S0-ANQ-634

On Your Terms

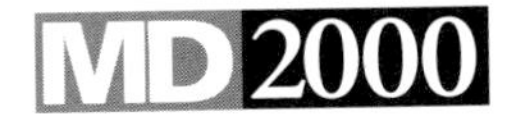

THE GRAND ROUNDS PRESS®

On Your Terms

Steven Gittelson

WHITTLE DIRECT BOOKS

The Grand Rounds Press: Dorothy Foltz-Gray, Editor;
Ken Smith, Design Director; Susan Brill, Art Director

Library of Congress Catalog Card Number: 94-60157
Gittelson, Steven
On Your Terms
ISBN 1-879736-22-5
ISSN 1053-6620

The Grand Rounds Press

The Grand Rounds Press publishes original short books by distinguished authors on subjects of importance to the medical profession. This year Grand Rounds presents MD/2000, a special series of four books designed to help doctors make sense of the rapid changes occurring in the U.S. health care delivery system.

Grand Rounds Press books, which appear approximately every three months, are edited and published by Whittle Books, a business unit of Whittle Communications L.P. They reflect a broad spectrum of responsible opinions. In each book the opinions expressed are those of the author, not the publisher or advertiser.

I welcome your comments on this unique endeavor.

William S. Rukeyser
Editor in Chief

For Elise
and
for my mother and father and sister

Acknowledgments

This book could not have been written without the cooperation, patience, and faith of a number of people. I deeply appreciate the time and courtesy of those who pointed me in the right direction, including Bette Waddington, a consultant with the Medical Group Management Association, Dr. Lane France, Dr. David Hubbard, Dr. Charlie Mercer, Patrick Patterson, vice-president of special projects at Health Midwest, and Grant Savage, professor of management at Texas Tech University. I am indebted to Pam Williams, whose research assistance enabled this project to be completed on time, and to Barbara Roberts, for smoothing out the kinks. I'll forever be grateful to my editor, Dorothy Foltz-Gray, for her unflagging support and patience. My deepest gratitude goes to my wife, Elise, whose ideas improved my manuscript, whose encouragement sustained me, whose faith in me exceeds my own.

contents

He published four volumes,
but he's best known for two words.

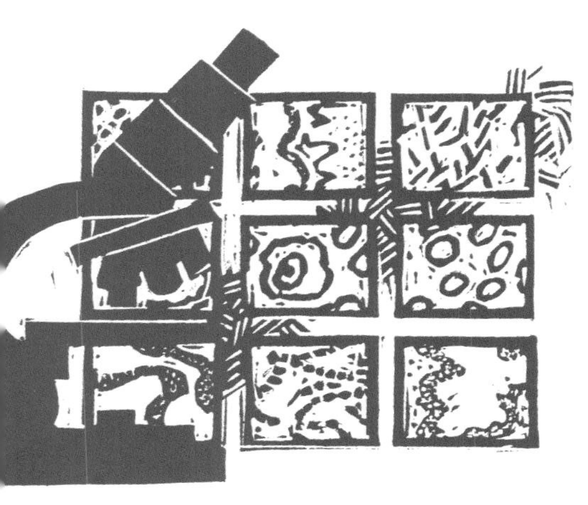

Miles is proud to present this series on...

Powerful Innovators

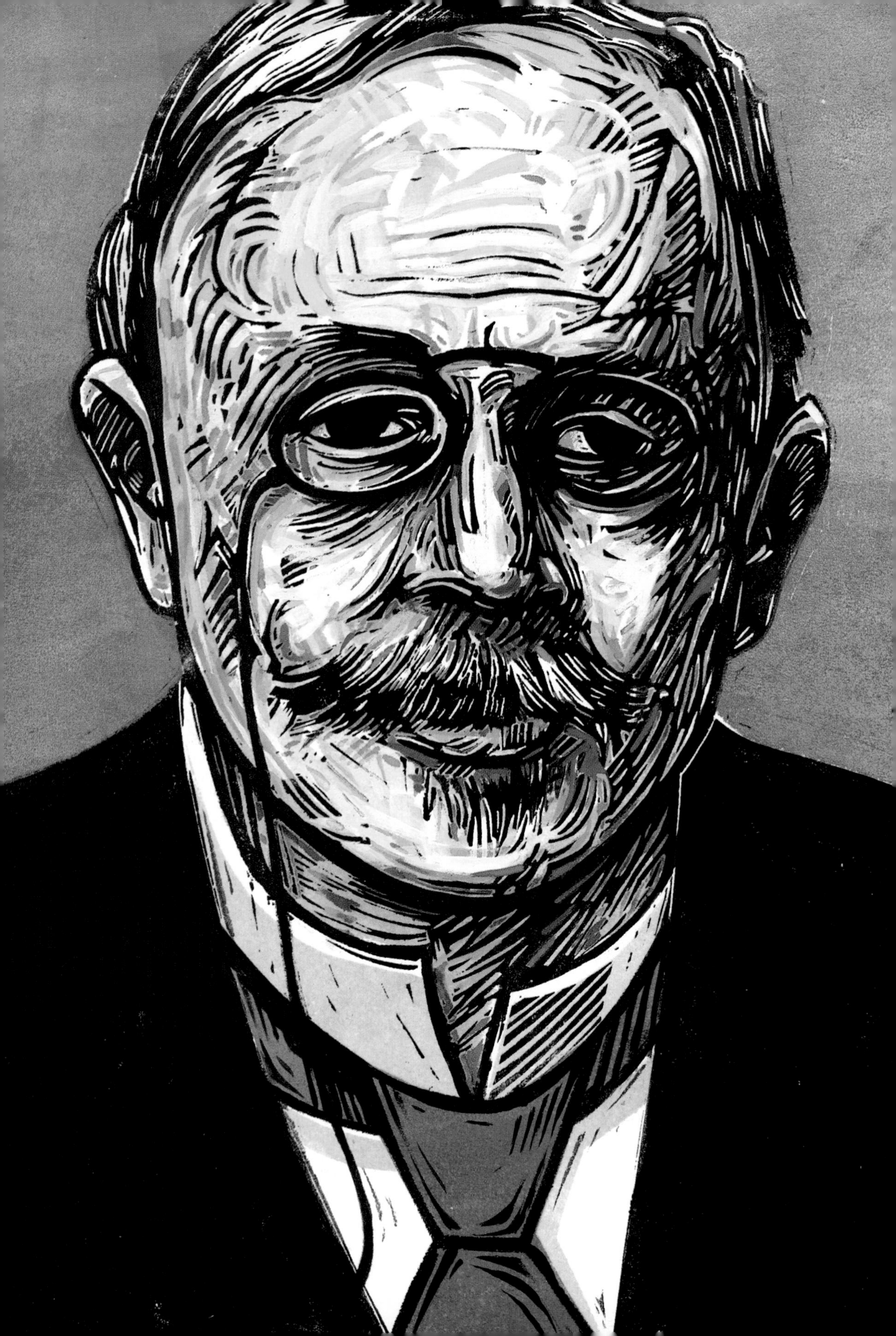

Powerful Physician

'ans Christian Joachim Gram (1853-1938)

The words "Gram's stain" are familiar to all physicians, but few know of the man behind the method.

A native of Copenhagen, Gram earned his medical degree at its University, then traveled in Europe, studying pharmacology and bacteriology.

In 1884, while working in Berlin, he published a paper describing his now-famous microbiologic staining method. While his technique was derived from Paul Ehrlich's staining of the tubercle bacillus, Gram's method proved applicable to all bacteria.

Gram returned to Copenhagen, where he became a popular professor and physician, and published a four-volume work on rational pharmacotherapy in clinical science. But his most significant work had already been done: the Gram method remains a first step in classifying and identifying bacteria, as well as assisting in determining the treatment of bacterial diseases.

Powerful Antimicrobial

Speed...power...efficacy against urinary tract infections, whatever the severity, and efficacy against mild to moderate lower respiratory and skin and skin structure infections.* That's the power of Cipro® I.V. The power that can make the difference in your practice.*

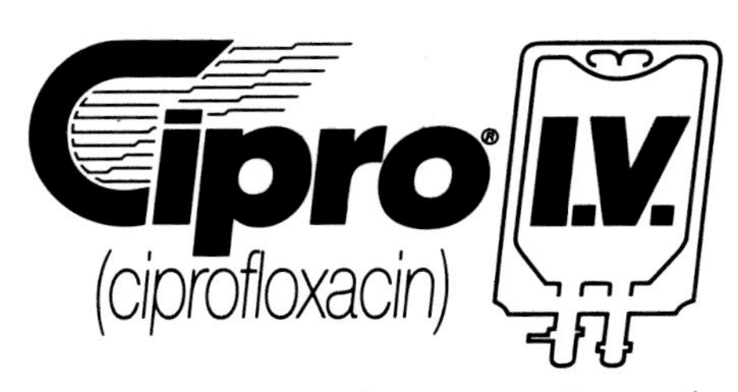

The most potent fluoroquinolone.[1-3†]

*Due to susceptible strains of indicated pathogens. See indicated organisms and dosage and administration sections in complete prescribing information.

†*In vitro* activity does not necessarily imply a correlation with *in vivo* results.

Please see complete prescribing information and cited references at the end of this book.

Powerful Numbers

speak for themselves:

***100**...Percent of patients whose severe urinary tract infections* resolved or improved† after 5.6 days of Cipro® I.V. therapy‡ in a recent Multicenter Study.*[4]

***95**...Percent of patients whose mild to moderate respiratory tract infections* resolved or improved† after 6.6 days of Cipro® I.V. therapy‡ in a recent Multicenter Study.*[4]

***95**...Percent of patients whose mild to moderate skin and skin structure infections* resolved or improved† after 7.2 days of Cipro® I.V. therapy‡ in a recent Multicenter Study.*[4]

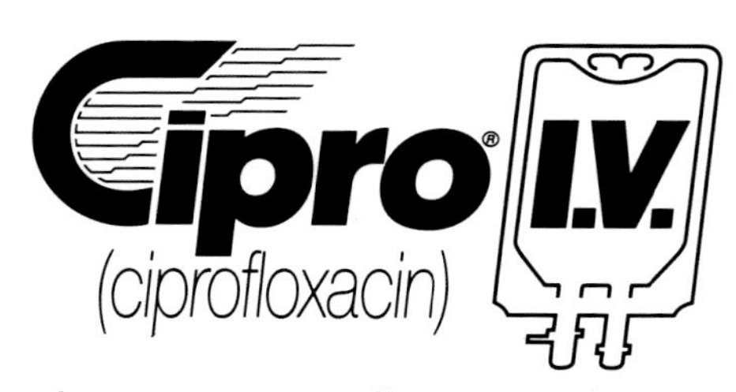

The most potent fluoroquinolone.[1-3§]

Please see complete prescribing information and cited references at the end of this book.

*In clinical studies, the most frequen
reported events, without regard to
relationship, among patients treate
with intravenous ciprofloxacin wer
nausea, diarrhea, central nervous s
disturbance, local iv site reactions,
abnormalities of liver associated en
(hepatic enzymes), and eosinophili
Headache, restlessness, and rash we
noted in greater than 1% of patien
treated with the most common dose
ciprofloxacin.*

*Due to susceptible strains of indicated pathogens. See ind
organisms and dosage and administration sections
complete prescribing information.

†Clinical response at the end of I.V. therapy (400 r
q12h). "Resolution" defined as disappearance or s
reduction of all signs and symptoms of infection t
discontinuance of antimicrobial therapy; "improv
defined as reduction in severity/number of signs a
symptoms, but requiring continued antimicrobial
Most "improved" patients were then switched to
oral therapy. Resolutions at posttreatment evaluat
were 85.3% for lower respiratory infections, 92.9
urinary tract infections, and 92.9% for skin and s
structure infections.

‡Average duration of Cipro® I.V. therapy.

§*In vitro* activity does not necessarily imply a correl
with *in vivo* results.

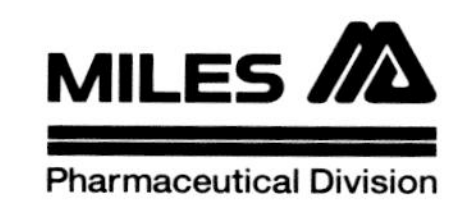

Miles Inc.
Pharmaceutical Divisior
400 Morgan Lane
West Haven, CT 06516

introduction

In Chicago an internist and an ophthalmologist negotiate a deal: the internist will refer his HMO patients who need cataract surgery to the specialist—if the procedure can be done for the right price. In Atlanta an allergist tells his competitors that financial ruin is imminent unless they form a network to win contracts from the managed-care plans. In California a family practitioner merges with a group of eight primary-care doctors because she desperately needs resources to deal with the 1,000 prepaid patients who have flooded her solo practice. In Minnesota several huge clinics are poised to grab the market away from 30 physicians in a multispecialty group that has served the residents of rural communities for three decades. To survive, the doctors sell their practice to a 500-physician university hospital complex, which also fears it is too small to compete in a turbulent medical marketplace.

Across the country primary-care physicians and specialists, in solo practices and in large groups, are struggling to save their careers. The spread of managed care and the specter of legislative reform have hit physicians like a right jab to the midsection followed by a left hook to the head. Those who were unprepared are stunned and embittered by the speed and severity of the assault.

The principal message for anyone practicing medicine in the 1990s is this: the changes rocking the profession require doctors to think like business owners. Patients are, after all, consumers of medical care, and their buying habits are changing. More than 45 million of them are enrolled in HMOs, and another 60 million subscribe to other types of managed-care plans. The only physicians who can treat them are those who enter the world of contract medicine. Understanding how managed-care contracts work—and what traps lie hidden within their legalese—is essential.

Merely being familiar with contract clauses, however, is no assurance that you will get the specific terms you want. To do that you need to know the fundamentals of negotiation, a skill physicians have never had to develop until now. And even sharpened negotiating skills will do little good unless you have some leverage. Many physicians feel intimidated by the prospect of going toe-to-toe with behemoth health plans, but they can strengthen their position if they understand what these outfits are looking for. Doctors who provide high-quality care and control costs already have distinguished themselves from their competition. And physicians who know how to lower their overheads, managing their practices as economically as any well-run business, are in a good position to handle the risks that come with treating prepaid patients.

Despite the profession's best lobbying efforts, managed-care organizations have been allowed to choose which physicians will be on their panels. This selectivity forces physicians to market themselves to the plans, another basic business skill that doctors have never before needed. The harsh reality for a profession formerly characterized by autonomy and independence is that managed-care organizations want to deal with groups of providers, not individuals. This fact, coupled with the uncertainties of pending health care reforms, is propelling physicians to consolidate at a frenetic pace. Solo practitioners are merging into groups. Medical groups are merging with one another. Large multispecialty groups are selling their practices to a variety of buyers, some of whom are traditional purchasers, some new to the scene. Understanding how these mergers work has now become vital to any physician who wants to remain competitive.

The most critical aspect of any type of consolidation maneuver is the ability to distinguish the right deal from the most lucrative deal. Knowing how to structure the arrangement so that you don't lose control over the way you practice medicine is a key strategic goal. Affiliating with an entity that's likely to be around for a while is another.

The ground is shaking and change is commonplace. These are not conditions anyone welcomes; they are distractions from healing the sick. But those who take the time to understand the dynamics that are reshaping the profession and acquire the strategic skills to negotiate their way through the turbulence will be well situated to return to the real business of medicine.

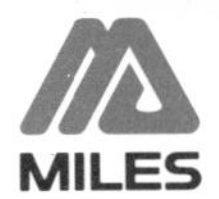

Miles Inc.
Pharmaceutical Division
400 Morgan Lane
West Haven, CT 06516

Edward L. Wilkerson
1464 E 105th St.
Cleveland, OH 44106-1100

Dear Doctor Wilkerson:

The healthcare system is moving towards managed care. Of this, there is no doubt. To navigate the sea of change, we must equip ourselves with a guide to survival. *On Your Terms*, the latest book from Grand Rounds Press, is just that.

In *On Your Terms*, the third of a four-volume series called *MD/2000*, Steve Gittleson discusses the legal and financial implications of managed care contracting, practice integration, and networking. Mr. Gittleson also explains the investigative, management, and negotiating skills that are crucial to physicians' survival in the revamped system.

Brought to you by Miles Inc., Pharmaceutical Division, maker of Cipro® (ciprofloxacin HCl) Tablets, *On Your Terms* also points out pitfalls that must be avoided and provides a plethora of examples and legal advice on how physicians can successfully meet the challenges of the reforming system.

We hope you find this book to be enjoyable.

Sincerely,

H. Brian Allen, M.D., FFPM
Director, Scientific Relations

SRG-0086005

CHAPTER *one*

SIZING UP THE PLANS

If fee-for-service medicine still reigned, Dr. David E. Nicklin would not be smiling. As a family-practice physician, he'd sit low on the medical totem pole, in both income and stature. And since one-quarter of his inner-city practice consists of welfare patients, the 39-year-old Philadelphian would probably be strapped as well; at $17 per office visit, Nicklin's Medicaid reimbursements would hardly cover his costs. Add to those low fees the uncollected ones from carriers that insure his other patients, and Nicklin would face a rising overhead coupled with a flat income.

That's the situation Nicklin faced in 1987 when he opened his doors. In 1994, however, he presides over a bustling practice. His capitated patient load has doubled to 6,000 in the past two years. To treat so many new patients, he has hired a staff that includes two full-time family-practice physicians, two physician assistants, and a nurse practitioner. And he has eliminated billing for 80 percent of his patients; instead, a predictable amount of cash flows into the office each month. What's more, a local hospital is poised to buy the practice for an amount he would only describe as greater than he'd ever dreamed possible. Thanks to a half-dozen capitated contracts with managed-care organizations—and his acumen as a physician—Nicklin couldn't be happier about practicing medicine in the 1990s.

Not all physicians share Nicklin's enthusiasm. For some, managed care equals mangled care. They fear, among other things, a loss of autonomy accompanied by a drop in income. Indeed, those nightmarish visions have come true for a number of physicians. No wonder much of the medical community has spent the past decade grieving over the approach of managed care. Many have denounced it as a fad; others have simply resigned themselves to change.

Doctors don't have to believe that managed care is the best thing since penicillin. But more than 100 million Americans are covered by managed-care plans, so physicians would be wise to accept the change as an inescapable reality. Acceptance means not only understanding how managed care works but developing skills that will enable doctors to benefit from the new order. The chief skill, as an increasing number of physicians can testify, is knowing how to contract with a managed-care organization. Unfortunately medical training has not equipped them for this challenge, and most doctors would rather dispense with contracts and the negotiations required to hammer them out. They just want to practice medicine. But unless they work in one of the few areas of the country where managed care has not yet surfaced, they cannot afford to neglect this skill, even temporarily.

As doctors contract with managed-care organizations, they will begin to run their practices more like service businesses. That won't be an easy transition, but they have little choice. Spiraling inflation in health care has eroded the loyalty patients once had to their physicians. Nowadays doctors must think of their patients as customers, consumers of medical services who are looking for the highest-quality care at the lowest price. Regardless of your diagnostic or clinical expertise, if 25 percent of the people in your community enroll in managed-care plans and you have no contracts with those plans, you have lost access to a quarter of your potential customers. How many companies can afford to write off that much business?

In addition to thinking of patients as customers, doctors are now forced to view their communities as markets. Before signing a contract or even deciding what provisions it should contain, physicians must determine the local level of managed care.

Managed care is spreading erratically. It dominates in some states, such as California and Minnesota, yet it's barely visible in the rural South and much of the Great Plains. State and local medical societies should be able to give you a good idea of just how rapidly managed care is spreading in your back yard—and it wouldn't hurt to update that information every three months or so. Other sources of information include local physicians, the managed-care directors of nearby hospitals, and the area's major employers.

Unfortunately no magic number or level of market penetration can serve as a signal to hop aboard the managed-care bandwagon. But this much is certain: although managed care grew slowly in its initial markets, it now spreads like kudzu once it hits town—in enrollees and in the types of contractual arrangements it offers.

In the many places where managed-care plans are establishing beachheads, HMOs and PPOs are inundating physicians with offers. This contracting frenzy and its profound economic impact on doctors has not been lost on the American Medical Association, which has hardly been a champion of managed care. Until recently it referred to the industry disapprovingly as an "alternative delivery system." No more. According to a 1993 report issued by its Center for Health Policy Research, even the AMA acknowledges that "the characterization of these relationships as 'alternative' arrangements may be outdated." Seventy percent of all physicians are involved with managed care, according to the report, and "half of all contracting physicians derive between 10 percent and 50 percent of their revenue from contracts."

Despite the plans' come-hither winks, a prudent first step for physicians is to suppress any impulse to sign up with all players. Some outfits are solvent, others are not. Some are in trouble with regulators, others are not. Some may follow sound policies regarding utilization, others may not. When it comes to checking out a managed-care plan, there are no shortcuts. Time is a physician's most precious commodity, but a few hours of research about any plan you may join could prevent disaster later on.

How can you size up an organization? If the plan is new in town, find out whether it's owned by a major national company or backed by the same folks who sold you your car. If it has been operating for a while, call some participating physicians to find out about their experiences. In either case, the organization's literature will probably answer some basic questions: Who are the top managers? Do physicians sit on the board? What is the medical director's background? Is the organization profitable? What is its current market share? What are its growth projections? How many group contracts does it have? What types of managed care is it offering? Who performs the utilization review and what criteria do they apply? What are the financial rewards of keeping utilization low? How and when are doctors reimbursed? Is the organization federally qualified? Is it accredited by an independent review board such as the National Committee for Quality Assurance, a 14-member board representing consumers, purchasers, providers of health care, and labor representatives?

Once you have reviewed the literature, get a sense of the group's values by calling the medical director and asking about the organization's policies and goals. Ask what the turnover rate is for primary-care physicians and specialists. For a plan that has been operating for four or five years, the figure should not be higher than 5 percent. If the rate is two or three times that, the director's strategy is backfiring.

Many doctors, pressed for time and ambivalent about contracting with managed-care organizations in the first place, may think that such inquiries are all that's necessary. But the wise doctor knows that independent sources of information provide the most objective and useful data. For $60, for example, Dun & Bradstreet will supply a report on an organization's financial behavior, including whether it is paying suppliers on time. If the company's stationery vendors have to go to court to get paid, its physicians will too.

State health and insurance departments are another excellent source of information. Forty-seven states have passed legislation governing the operation of HMOs, and 25 states regulate PPOs. The laws vary regarding capital reserves and quality control. In most states the insurance department regulates the financial and consumer aspects of the organizations, and the health department covers quality of care and utilization. Particularly useful are the annual reports of managed-care organizations, which typically include audited financial statements, lists of providers, and summaries of customer complaints.

What financial indicators are the most meaningful? The company's administrative and operating costs should not exceed 10 to 15 percent of total expenses; if the figure is well above that, the company may be too generous to its staff. Medical costs should be no more than 85 percent of expenses; if the figure is 90 percent or more, the company is paying out too much, probably to hospitals and specialists, and that can dramatically shorten a plan's life expectancy.

Although insurance companies and groups of doctors are concocting new types of managed-care arrangements at a dizzying rate, the choice for most physicians includes two types of plans: PPOs and HMOs. Primary-care physicians who treat 2,000 or so patients in areas where managed care is well established sometimes contract with a half-dozen HMOs and 10 to 20 PPOs.

The arrangement a physician chooses depends on what's offered locally and how much economic risk he or she is willing to accept. Those who merely want to nibble at the table of managed care will opt for a preferred-provider organization, which links participating physicians and hospitals with employer groups or other buyers of health care. Doctors sign contracts negotiated on their behalf by the PPO, agreeing to accept 10 to 20 percent less than their normal fees, depending on the region and the bargaining abilities of the PPO. In return for the discounted fees, physicians hope to treat more patients.

It looks like a straightforward deal: physicians give up some revenue, and the PPO sells the physicians' services to its many subscribers. But to Jerry P. Clousson, a hard-nosed former labor lawyer who has spent 20 years representing physicians, no deal is ever as simple as it appears. "Look at what's really getting marketed in this situation," he said. "There is no plan without the physicians. The plan is using the doctor's name to market itself. And what does the physician get? As soon as he signs up, a certain percentage of his regular fee-for-service patients will sign up with the PPO, and the next time they see that physician, they'll be discounted patients. So the physician has lost some revenue right off the bat. And what's he got in return? Nothing." In a vacuum Clousson's comments are accurate, but given the medical market of the 1990s, what PPOs and HMOs offer is survival; that is, access to a growing population of patients.

Clousson, a Chicagoan and former head of the AMA's negotiating department, says doctors should think before they leap into any managed-care plan, especially one just getting off the ground. "There are only two reasons why a physician should want to join one," he said. "To protect or increase his market share—that means making sure the plan has a market share—and to ensure quick payment."

Since patients can choose any provider within a network, PPOs cannot guarantee physicians an increase in patients. So how can doctors improve the odds of benefiting from such an arrangement? In addition to inquiring about the number of subscribers in a PPO, doctors need to find out where those subscribers live. If the largest employer in town signs up with a PPO, the providers whose practices are either near the company's headquarters or in the suburbs where its employees live are most likely to gain patients. Doctors in outlying areas may see little or no increase.

Physicians have virtually no power to negotiate the discount down from, say, 20 percent to 15 or 10 percent. PPOs do not want the headache of administering a thousand different fee arrangements with as many doctors. Nonetheless a physician can figure out whether a deal is financially sound. First, if the PPO is several years old, ask participating doctors whether they receive payment within 30 days; they should not have to wait any longer. Second, review the PPO's list of covered medical services to make sure it includes the tasks you perform most frequently. Third, unless the PPO is owned by an outfit with deep pockets—an insurance company or a hospital—find out who has the ultimate responsibility for payment and whether that organization is solvent. This is critical, since a contract between a PPO and a doctor prohibits the physician from balance-billing, even if the PPO goes bankrupt.

Physicians who gain a lot of patients through PPOs should anticipate an increase in administrative hassles. According to David E. Vogel, a managed-care consultant to the AMA and author of *Family Physicians and Managed Care: A View to the 90s*, PPOs are more loosely structured than HMOs and provide little incentive for physicians to manage care more effectively than they have in the past. Many doctors, eager to make up revenue lost through discounted fees, compensate by ordering more tests and services, and that costs the PPOs more. The PPOs respond by tightening administrative controls such as utilization review and precertification. "This creates a certain amount of tension between some PPOs and their participating physicians," writes Vogel. For these reasons some managed-care experts deride PPOs as "transitional products."

Discounted fee-for-service medicine has two basic weaknesses: it has not effectively lowered the nation's health care costs, and it fails to make costs predictable to insurers and purchasers. HMOs try to skirt these problems by using the reimbursement method called capitation.

If capitation hasn't yet come to your neighborhood, it will, and sooner than you think. The marketplace is hurtling in this direction.

For the moment, most HMOs use capitation to reimburse primary-care physicians—family practitioners, general internists, and pediatricians—and use a discounted fee schedule to pay specialists. Staff-model, or closed-panel, HMOs pay physicians a straight salary.

Saying that capitation presents a challenge to primary-care physicians is like calling a marathon a runners' race; it doesn't begin to indicate the scope. The scariest aspect of capitation is that it reverses the traditional economics of a medical practice. In a fee-for-service practice, the more services performed, the greater the income. In a capitated system, the fewer the services per patient, the greater the income. The financial incentive therefore shifts to providing only what is absolutely necessary.

"To succeed, most physicians will have to change their traditional prescribing patterns," said Alice G. Gosfield, a health lawyer in Philadelphia and past president of the National Health Lawyers Association. "In a fee-for-service system, you maximize your reimbursement through overutilization," she said. "In this system, you maximize your reimbursement through underutilization. Where you draw the line is the great tension that exists in managed care. It hits physicians where they live."

Indeed, many physicians remain skeptical about managed care precisely because too many HMOs have drawn the line poorly; they have paid too much attention to controlling costs, too little to ensuring high-quality care. Although this balancing act is occurring with wildly uneven results throughout the HMO industry, the best-managed HMOs know that health care buyers want more than mere cost-containment. The message large employers are sending to insurers, Gosfield said, is that they are "interested in value—controlled costs and good outcomes for patients, as demonstrated by hard data."

Physicians, therefore, must learn where their local HMO has drawn its line between cost and care. Does its utilization-management system lower costs by eliminating only unnecessary care? Or does it deny some appropriate care? Does the plan oblige a doctor to provide only those services that ordinarily fall within his or her specialty? Or does it require primary-care physicians to perform procedures they normally don't do in order to save money on specialists?

Physicians must also know when they will need authorization for hospital admission, what the HMO's policy is regarding the length of hospitalization for various conditions, and what the organization considers a medical emergency. Unfortunately many HMOs do not allow physicians to review their utilization-management protocols, although the better-run plans are making such information available.

An HMO's utilization restrictions clearly affect how comfortable a doctor will be practicing medicine. Less obvious is the impact those policies have on professional liability. "Physicians are still liable for bad outcomes when they do not provide access to certain kinds of care," Gosfield said. This is critical for a primary-care physician who contracts with HMOs that require the doctor to act as a gatekeeper. According to Gosfield, even court rulings that have held plans liable have not exempted the affiliated physicians from liability.

Capitation also exposes a practice to economic risks. If too many patients require too much care, a physician could rapidly go bankrupt. On the other hand, rather than waiting two or more months for a patient or insurer to pay a bill, the doctor generally receives payments monthly for capitated patients. A healthy cash flow keeps suppliers happy, and the physician can park any surplus in an interest-bearing account. Perhaps the greatest blessing is that prepaid patients require no billing. Imagine not having to deal with dozens of different insurance forms. Better yet, imagine eliminating the "funds uncollected" column from your books.

It is impossible to determine whether an HMO's capitation rate is adequate unless the physician knows the specific medical services the rate covers and the demographics of the patient population. Under capitation, physicians are responsible for keeping the cost of care down with every treatment decision they make. So they need to know ahead of time precisely what the capitation fee covers. Does it include such services as lab work and X-rays? In many plans it does not.

In fee-for-service medicine, the nature of a patient's illness rarely has an adverse effect on a physician's income. The doctor gives the patient whatever treatment is needed, sends a bill, and collects a payment. But when a doctor is treating prepaid patients, that approach doesn't fly, because some patient groups require more care than others. HMOs realize this, and that's why their formulas for computing capitation rates are based on such factors as age and sex. Infants and toddlers under 2 may be assigned a rate of, say, $21 each per month. Those between the ages of 2 and 4 may have a rate of $11, between 5 and 20 a rate of $5, and over 21 a rate of $8. Women in their child-bearing years have a higher rate than men the same age. The HMO sorts its enrollees by demographic criteria, tabulates the numbers, and pays the physician what's called a blended, or single, rate.

Just as the HMO analyzes data so that it knows what to charge members and pay providers, so physicians must study the patient population. The core question is, what groups is the HMO targeting? Doctors can't determine whether a capitation rate is reasonable unless they can anticipate, at least in a general sense, their patients' probable medical needs. If the dominant employer in a community is a coal company, for example, it is important to know whether the local HMO intends to sign it up. Obviously those patients stand a better chance of contracting respiratory problems than people who work behind desks. There is no reason to shun an HMO that enrolls such members, but a doctor can't judge a capitation rate unless that fact is known up front. Similarly, if an HMO has a high proportion of members younger than 2 or older than 65, physicians can expect frequent office visits and hospitalizations.

"Trying to figure out a capitation rate with a new HMO is a crapshoot," said Clousson. "You never know what the mix of patients is going to be." If an HMO has been operating for a few years, assessing the capitation rate is easier. Talk to physicians who have experience with the HMO. Do they think the rate is reasonable for the population they serve?

Another critical issue is adverse selection. Flip a coin 10 times and it could land heads up seven or eight times. Flip the same coin 1,000 times and the odds improve enormously that heads and tails will be almost evenly split. Physicians who are timid about capitation might think it makes sense to see only 10 prepaid patients. Thanks to adverse selection, however, seven or eight of them could be ill, in which case the physician would spend hours treating them and lose money. But if a doctor sees the right number of patients, the risk of adverse selection disappears. According to most experts, a typical solo practice needs 200 to 300 prepaid patients per capitated account to minimize the risk of an excessively ill population.

Many doctors wonder what percentage of their practice should be devoted to managed care. One rule of thumb suggests that if X percent of the people in a community belong to managed-care plans, then area physicians should have roughly that percentage in their practices. Otherwise they are out of sync with the marketplace, and they could find themselves crowded out. To get the number of managed-care patients they're after, physicians generally need contracts with several HMOs and PPOs. Just as investing all of your money in a single stock is unwise, so is relying on one contract to generate the bulk of your revenue. "When you can't afford to lose that payer," said Clousson, "then you've become an economic slave."

Until a physician is used to the new economic system, gauging the adequacy of a capitation rate will be difficult. Some HMOs and PPOs complicate the process by penalizing physicians who fail to stay within budget and rewarding those who minimize testing, referrals, and hospital admissions. Some groups hold back part of the reimbursement, usually 20 percent. So doctors who have a blended capitation rate of $10 for each enrollee receive only $8 a month, and the plan deposits $2 in its "withhold" fund. If at the end of the year the doctors have exceeded the budget by ordering too many services, they lose the withheld funds. If the physicians have met the plan's financial goals, they get the money back. Withhold pools are unpopular among doctors, who grouse that sanctions are built into their reimbursements, so the more progressive HMOs have dropped this feature.

In place of withholds many HMOs use a friendlier approach to cost control. They pay physicians a capitation rate and add bonuses if the doctors hold referrals and hospitalizations in check. The bonuses come out of accounts called risk pools, funded by the HMOs. Some plans use one risk pool to pay specialists and hospital care; others use two separate pools. Some also award cash bonuses for sound management practices. The sum of these incentives can be substantial.

Consider the case of Dr. David Nicklin, the family-practice physician in Philadelphia. Unlike many of his peers, Nicklin is comfortable with managed care and chose to become involved with HMOs soon after he opened his practice in 1987. "It was an easy transition because we already were treating our people as outpatients if possible," he said. "I never believed in ordering CAT scans for every headache. Some folks act like [insurance money] is Monopoly money, but I never thought of it that way."

Nicklin and the two family-practice physicians he hired treat about 9,000 patients. Some 2,000 pay fees for service while the rest are en-

"I have worked as hard as I could... if my success has been greater than that of most...the reason is that I came in my wanderings through the medical field upon regions where the gold was still lying by the wayside...and that is of no great merit."

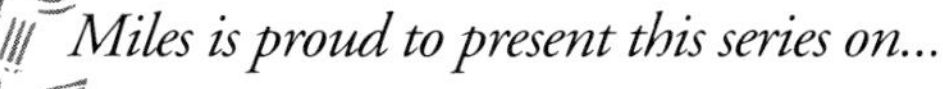

Miles is proud to present this series on...

Powerful Innovators

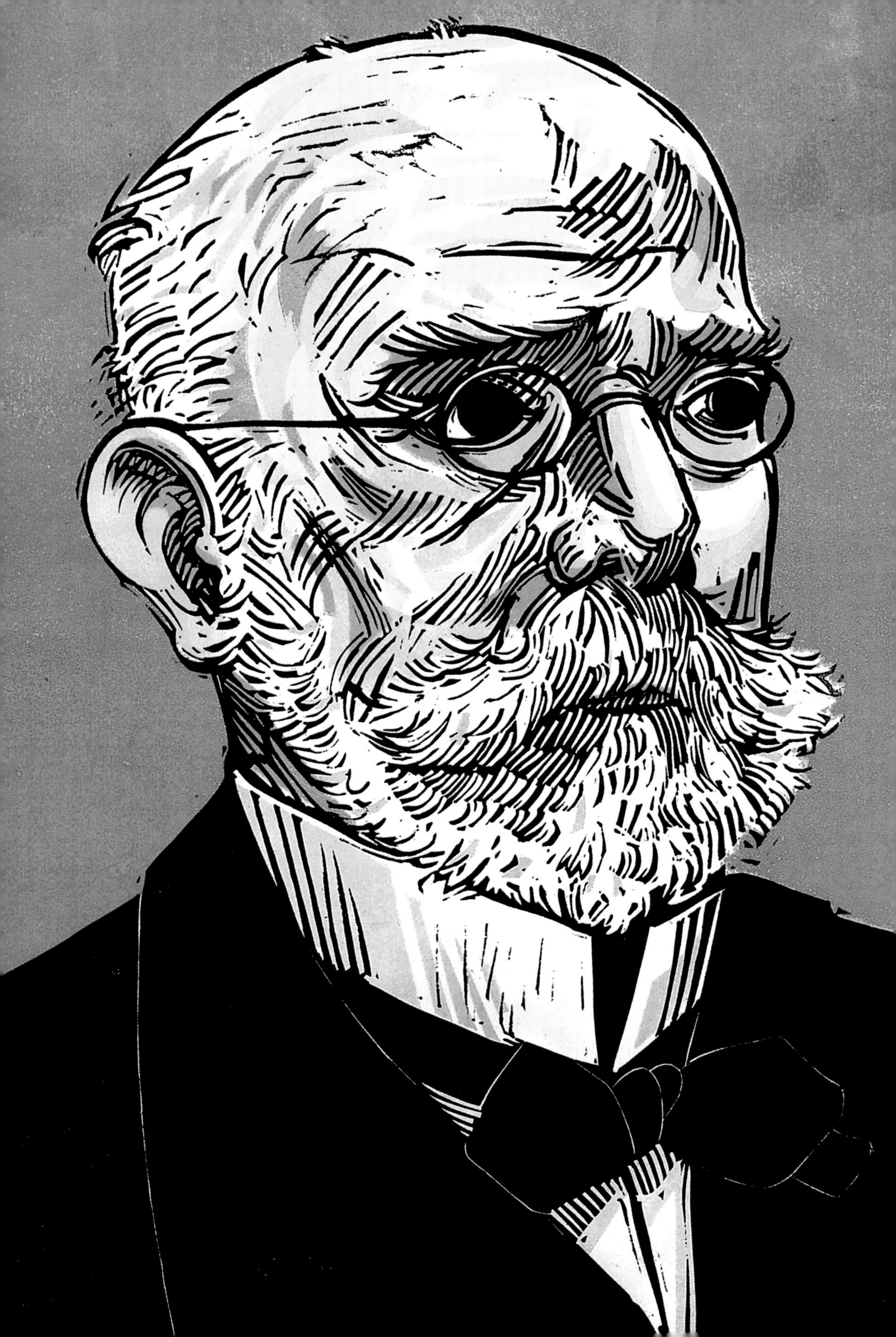

Powerful Physician

Robert Koch (1843-1910)

Even Koch himself would have been surprised to learn in 1866 that he would become one of the most important bacteriologists of all time. His dream of traveling to exotic ports took an ironic turn when his wife's gift of a microscope spurred his interest in the exotic world of microbes.

With a passionate interest in bacteriology generated by a crisis that struck in 1876 (an anthrax epidemic among local cattle), Koch studied the disease, cultured the organism on artificial media, analyzed its complete life cycle, and transferred the infection to mice.

Koch's research in bacteriology continued: He isolated and cultivated staphylococci from surgical infections, analyzed streptococci taken from wound exudate, and discovered the bacillus that causes conjunctivitis. Perhaps his most important contribution was the discovery of the bacillus responsible for tuberculosis, a devastating illness at that time.

rolled in one of six HMOs the practice contracts with. As he shopped for HMOs, Nicklin noticed that the capitation rates differed by as much as 30 percent. None had a withhold fund. "The less sophisticated HMOs offer a flat capitation rate with virtually no incentives, or else their rewards are based on the performance of all the doctors in the plan," Nicklin said. "The better ones offer handsome bonuses that are tied to the performance of individual practices."

Nicklin's practice typically receives a base capitation payment of $9 to $10 per month for each HMO patient. Add the incentives the practice receives and the figure jumps to $13. Since 6,000 patients are capitated, the incentives amount to at least $18,000 every month. "The bonus money represents the difference between making ends meet and being financially comfortable," he said.

How do Nicklin and his colleagues earn such an impressive bonus? The way the practice is managed accounts for about half of the extra dollars. The physicians receive bonus money for staying open three nights a week and every Saturday, for getting good grades on patient satisfaction surveys, and for having low patient turnover. Doctors who take continuing medical education courses receive additional bonuses, and two HMOs reward the practice for accepting new patients.

The other half of the bonus is a reward for minimizing tests and referrals. The group performs all the normal diagnostic tests and procedures of a primary-care office and treats uncomplicated dermatological, orthopedic, and urological complaints. Most blood work and all X-rays are done by specialists. "My practice pattern hasn't changed. I've always practiced cost-effective medicine," said Nicklin. If a patient complains of chest pain, for example, Nicklin advises him or her to come in for an EKG instead of immediately involving a cardiologist. "Managed-care plans do well because they control costs," he said. "As a doctor contracting with managed-care plans, I do the same."

The plans don't micromanage Nicklin's practice or hassle him about referrals to specialists. And precertification for hospitalization hasn't changed either; he uses the same process he has always used with indemnity insurers. "No one has run me around asking whether the clinical care I provide is necessary," he said.

Since 1992 the HMOs have doubled the number of patients Nicklin sees. He concedes that prepaid patients make more appointments than fee-for-service ones. To ease the strain on the three-doctor staff,

Nicklin hired two physician assistants and a nurse practitioner. "I recommend hiring that kind of help when your practice swells in size," he said. The salary of a nurse practitioner is about half of a physician's. "Our nurse sees as many patients as a doctor, and the patients are happy with the arrangement," said Nicklin, "as long as they're seen on time and the work gets done properly."

Primary-care doctors with multiple HMO contracts should monitor their results every quarter. Nicklin evaluates how much each plan pays him, how many patients each sends him, and how many office visits the patients schedule. Periodically scrutinizing the numbers tells him which HMOs bring him money and which ones drain it away. "It's an important mechanism for primary-care physicians who have prepaid patients," he said. Nicklin also suggests that doctors compare the reimbursements from monthly capitated services with the practice's normal charges. He charges $30 to $40 for a routine follow-up office visit, for example. He calculates that the same visit earns him $10 to $20 more under capitation, including bonus dollars.

Studying the numbers may be a headache, but Nicklin has few complaints. About 80 percent of his patients require no billing. The average reimbursement per patient visit from one HMO, thanks to a generous incentive program, is $64. Another HMO pays an average of $50 per patient visit. Nicklin's 1,400 welfare patients—for whom Medicaid paid him $17 per visit—are now enrolled in an HMO that reimburses him an average of $52 per visit.

"Frankly, my practice couldn't exist in its current form in this location if we were operating in a fee-for-service universe," said Nicklin. "The patients who come here are working people. If they had to pay $50 a visit every time they walked in the door, the volume would drop off dramatically, and my uncollected accounts would rise astronomically. The fee-for-service model may work in affluent suburbs where patients have major medical and get 80 percent of their money refunded, but it sure doesn't work in neighborhoods like mine."

Besides understanding reimbursement systems, doctors have to decipher the provisions of contracts that address issues like termination rights, indemnification, and exclusivity. Since capitation is a dicier game than discounted fees, HMO contracts merit close scrutiny.

Doctors are not used to practicing medicine by contract, and since they're usually pressed for time, some might be inclined to read an agreement too quickly. They should keep these warnings in mind: First, a lawyer representing the interests of the managed-care organization wrote the contract; it favors the organization, not the physician. Second, poorly written contracts contain vague words such as *may*, *when necessary*, or *when appropriate*; make sure these terms are defined. As with any business contract, have a lawyer review the document before you sign it. It's best to hire one who is familiar with managed-care contracts, since health law is a specialized field. An increasing number of state medical societies provide this service.

A key provision in any contract is the one that explains how the parties can bail out if the deal backfires. No physician should sign up with a PPO or an HMO without understanding the rules for terminating the agreement. Generally either the physician or the managed-care company can terminate the contract "with cause" or "without cause." Most managed-care contracts contain clauses allowing either party to end the agreement without cause following 60 or 90 days' notice. This provision benefits the plan, said attorney Alice Gosfield, because "managed-care plans routinely engage in economic credentialing." That is, they determine which doctors have the highest costs and proceed to fire them. In the business world it's called downsizing. Since a physician can be fired at any time, financial security is an illusion. The only good news, said Gosfield, is that organizations that terminate a physician without cause may not report the action to the National Practitioner Data Bank, a service within the Department of Health and Human Services that provides a kind of professional background check on physicians and other health professionals. In certain instances a payer may report a termination with cause, so make sure the contract lists the precise circumstances under which the plan can dismiss you with cause—if your license were suspended, for instance, or if you lost your hospital privileges.

A physician can attempt to even the balance of power by asking the plan to remove the "without cause" provision after the first year. Another strategy is to change the notice period from 60 or 90 days to six or nine months, which at least cushions the blow. However, if a physician wants to terminate the agreement with cause—which might arise, for example, if the plan fails to pay its reimbursements—six or nine months' notice is too long. In that situation, the less time the better.

Another potential minefield for physicians is the standard "hold harmless" indemnification clause found in many contracts. According to *Evaluating Managed Care Contracts*, published by the American Academy of Pediatrics, health plans view physicians as independent contractors: "In the event of a medical liability action, a contract that contains a 'hold harmless' clause states that the plan . . . is free from any liability as a result of the physician's action and renders the physician solely responsible for damages." Health care lawyers say physicians simply should not sign a contract that contains this provision. In some states, in fact, malpractice carriers will not allow physicians they insure to agree to it. Managed-care organizations routinely stick the clause in their contracts and just as routinely remove it if a physician objects.

Some contracts disguise the issue by stating that "all medical decisions are rendered solely by independent contracting physicians and not by the HMO." Surely if a patient enrolled in an HMO is harmed as a result of tight medical restrictions, the HMO should be held at least partially responsible. Indeed, several courts have ruled that an HMO and its contracted doctors—much like a hospital and its physicians—both have legal responsibilities for the delivery of medical care.

What can happen if a physician unwittingly indemnifies an HMO? Say a patient files a malpractice suit naming both parties as codefendants. Even if a judge dismisses the suit, the HMO could force the physician to pay its legal bills. Worse yet, if the case is settled or lost at trial, the doctor would have to pay all damages. And since many malpractice insurers do not cover risk assumed under an indemnity clause, little would stand between the physician and financial ruin.

Beware, too, of contracts that contain exclusivity clauses, which bar a physician from contracting with other managed-care plans in the community. As noted earlier, primary-care physicians need multiple managed-care contracts to avoid economic enslavement.

Another contract component that has significance for physicians is the stop-loss provision. Managed-care plans buy stop-loss "reinsurance"—insurance to protect themselves against catastrophic medical expenses. The contract should also protect physicians from personal financial harm by including a stop-loss ceiling, which might be $3,000 to $5,000 per physician in a small practice.

A contract also spells out how a plan handles its risk-pool funds. Since these accounts, which pay for services such as specialists and inpatient care, can add tens of thousands of dollars annually to a primary-care doctor's base capitation, it is important to note the terms precisely. Look for a specific list of services the funds cover. The contract should also specify how the plan calculates surpluses and when they are distributed. Although it's uncommon, a contract could require a physician to pay the plan if the risk pool runs a deficit. Helping the HMO pay for its budgetary miscalculation could prove costly; the smart preemptive move would be to limit the dollar amount a doctor would have to pay.

Some contracts also include one or more attached documents. A doctor cannot afford to ignore such exhibits, which carry as much legal weight as the clauses in the body of the boilerplate contract. These attachments may list the medical services a physician is obligated to provide and the organization's utilization-review protocols. Packaging a contract this way makes it easier for a plan to change some of its fundamental components. Most managed-care contracts give the organization the right to unilaterally amend its policies, and such changes are often in the exhibits. A physician can't do much about exhibits other than request several months' notice before the plan implements any policy changes—or ink in a clause voiding the agreement if the plan proposes truly substantial changes.

Since HMOs can change their policies at any time, physicians have nothing to gain by asking for long-term contracts. Most contracts last one year and renew automatically unless either party terminates them. Gosfield calls them "Energizer bunny contracts" because they just keep going and going. She adds that the duration of an agreement becomes meaningless if the plan is allowed to dismiss a physician without cause in 60 or 90 days. In that situation the physician has, in effect, a 60- or 90-day contract.

If sizing up managed-care plans, analyzing capitation rates, and sorting through contractual legalese sounds complicated and time-consuming, that's because it is. Yet these are merely the basics of managed-care contracting. Understanding how capitation works doesn't necessarily mean you will get the rates you want, and the ability to spot disadvantageous clauses in a plan's contract isn't worth a lot unless you can alter them. The art of managed-care contracting also involves knowing whether you possess the clout to get what you want and using that leverage effectively.

CHAPTER *two*

NEGOTIATIONS: YOUR CLOUT AND THEIRS

The AMA isn't ahead of the curve on many issues these days, says Chicago health lawyer Jerry Clousson, but in the mid-1970s the organization foresaw the arrival of what it dubbed "contract medicine." Sensing that big changes were about to rock the profession, the AMA hired Clousson to teach the fundamentals of negotiating to medical societies.

"When I'd talk to these doctors about negotiating, they'd laugh," said Clousson. "They'd say, 'Negotiate? Negotiate with whom? What on earth are you talking about?'"

Twenty years later, teaching physicians how to negotiate has become a multimillion-dollar business. The doctor-as-student has money in hand and a need to learn as much as possible as quickly as possible; it's no wonder entrepreneurs are approaching physicians the way hungry tigers approach baby antelope. If you call your local medical society, the chances are good that during any given month it is sponsoring at least one workshop devoted to contract negotiations. And the AMA offers a slickly packaged nine-part series on managed care and contracting that includes videotapes, audiocassettes, and pamphlets.

Until the mid-1980s health care lawyers and consultants generally worked the managed-care organizations' side of the table because that's where the business was; now they are selling their services to doctors. Simply because someone has spent most of his or her time advising health plans instead of doctors, however, does not necessarily mean the guidance is suspect. In fact, said Alice Gosfield, "sometimes it's very useful to have somebody who comes from the plan perspective telling you how you stack up against your peers, rather than somebody who's going to put a ball of sunshine in your ear." Just make sure you know which side of the table an adviser on managed care favors.

It is not surprising that so many physicians are scrambling to learn about contracting with HMOs. The effect managed care has on the medical profession is similar to the power that a phonograph has in a game of musical chairs. In many cities the music is fading and the players are nervously eyeing the available chairs. "The big message," said Gosfield, "is that not everybody can continue to play."

To understand what Gosfield means, simply examine the life cycle of a managed-care plan. When an HMO comes to town, its arms are open. It spends its childhood busily marketing itself to health care purchasers and to the doctors who will offer care. In its adolescence it continues growing and starts collecting data on all its physicians—the number of tests each one orders, the number of times each sends a patient to a specialist or a hospital, and so forth. The HMO reaches adulthood when it has gained as much market share as possible in a community. At that point, since few new patient groups remain, revenues plateau. But to satisfy owners or shareholders, profits must keep growing. The HMO uses the data it has collected to create economic profiles of its providers; the ones who cost the plan the most are not invited to renew their contracts. The HMO decides that the remaining physicians are sufficient to treat the plan's members. No new doctors need apply.

Private-practice physicians already face this worrisome situation in Southern California, Portland, Oregon, the Twin Cities in Minnesota, Albuquerque, Seattle, and many other places where managed care is entrenched. Moreover, HMOs founded in the 1970s and '80s took a decade or more to evolve from infancy to adulthood; in the 1990s it takes just a few years. Physicians who turn their backs on managed care until they begin to lose patients risk being shut out of the marketplace altogether.

To counter this trend some medical associations are lobbying for states to pass "any willing provider" legislation, which would require managed-care plans to contract with any physician willing to abide by the plans' rules. Supporters say such laws are needed to give doctors access to patients and to ensure patients' freedom in choosing a physician. Opponents claim the measures' intent is to stop the plans from selective contracting, which is how managed-care plans contain costs. As of 1994 the AMA's success has been marginal. Since 1989 15 states have passed such measures in various watered-down forms; in seven of those states, for example, the law applies only to pharmacists. The prognosis for relief seems dim: the Department of Justice and the Federal Trade Commission oppose the legislation.

Some doctors understandably feel as though they're in front of a steamroller, powerless to halt its progress and intimidated by the size of the machine. However, managed-care organizations are businesses that act in predictable ways and value certain types of physicians more than others. Once you know how HMOs behave, striking a deal on your terms is much easier.

What an HMO values depends on local market conditions. In cities where HMOs have a stranglehold on health care—"mature markets," in the argot of consultants—the best opportunities for physicians are in outlying suburbs. These HMOs expand market share by reaching deep into the bedroom communities where commuters live. Since people aren't likely to sign up with doctors who are more than 20 to 30 minutes away, managed-care plans need providers who live near their new members. Doctors in such areas are literally well-positioned to win favorable contracts.

"The first thing doctors have to do to negotiate effectively," said Clousson, "is to understand their position in the marketplace and to perceive their strengths and weaknesses." This is particularly true in less developed managed-care markets, where HMOs are still attempting to cover a metropolitan area and the most densely populated adjacent suburbs. In a sense this less mature market provides the best deal for physicians. The plans are growing at a healthy clip, so they need more providers. Moreover, they have been operating for a while, and that makes it relatively easy for doctors to see how they are run, whether they have a good mix of members, and whether they have been able to attract high-caliber physicians and hospitals.

Physicians' ability to strike a good deal in this type of market depends on where they sit on the medical totem pole. In the eyes of managed-care organizations, solo practitioners occupy the lowest position whereas large multispecialty clinics sit at the top. Just as health insurers prefer to sign up large groups of patients rather than individuals, they prefer to work with teams of providers rather than solo physicians. Administratively it is much easier to deal with groups, and the more services a group offers and the larger the geographic area it covers, the better. A doctor's leverage increases proportionately as he or she moves up the pole.

More important than a practice's location or size, however, is the physician's attitude toward managed care. The doctors who are most appealing to an HMO are those who can demonstrate clinical skill combined with a commitment to cost control. The thought of marketing themselves makes many physicians uncomfortable, but that time-honored sensibility can be a liability in the new medical marketplace. The world of contract medicine rewards those who are assertive, who step forward to tell an HMO medical director that the concept of managed care is not really so radical because they themselves have been delivering quality care in an efficient manner throughout their careers. They may be obstetricians who perform fewer C-sections than their peers, or internists who treat more conditions on an outpatient basis than their colleagues. They know their economic and clinical profiles: their patients spend fewer days in the hospital than average and have better outcomes. Now they are speaking the HMO's language.

A physician's marketing approach might also include something as seemingly trivial as patient-satisfaction surveys. The notion of sampling customers' opinions may seem more appropriate for a car dealership or a telephone company. But many HMOs place a high value on customer satisfaction, and physicians who can show that their practices score well stand a better chance of negotiating a good deal than those who scoff at such measures. "There are two ways to get a good negotiating position with managed-care plans," said Dr. Joel I. Shalowitz, an internist and director of the Health Services Management Program at Northwestern University's J.L. Kellogg Graduate School of Management. "Number one, you can be the only group in the area, which gives you instant power. Number two, you can provide good-quality care—medical quality and service quality." Is service truly so significant? "Absolutely," Shalowitz said. "There are a lot of good doctors around, but not a lot of well-managed practices. Service is an issue of strategic importance to any group that wants to succeed in this environment."

This news may make many doctors sick at heart, including a primary-care physician I know. More often than not one of this fellow's patients could practically read *War and Peace* by the time his name is called. Arguments among nurses and receptionists ricochet off the waiting-room walls. In short, the management of the practice is abysmal. Yet the patients keep returning because the doctor is a gifted diagnostician who spends as much time as it takes to pinpoint a problem. How would such a doctor fare in this new environment? He wouldn't make it, concluded several consultants. His clinical expertise would not outweigh his poor management skills, and an HMO would probably release him.

For better or worse, doctors who once thought that providing superior medical care was all that mattered now find their practices judged by the same criteria consumers use to evaluate any service business: Is the staff friendly, helpful, informed, and efficient? Is the office pleasant-looking and conveniently located? Are complaints resolved courteously and quickly? This is just another way in which the world of contract medicine requires physicians to think of their practices as businesses. Those who see these road signs and follow them have a significant advantage over their competitors when negotiating with HMOs.

The surest way a physician can win better terms than those in a boilerplate managed-care contract is to view the contracting organization as a business partner, not an enemy. If doctors can help an organization operate more effectively, they can gain an equal footing with their negotiating partner. "Negotiation is a very realistic exercise," Clousson said. "If I need you, I'll negotiate with you. If I don't need you, I won't."

True negotiations only occur between parties that are roughly equal in power. Mere equality, however, doesn't automatically secure the agreement you want. To succeed in any type of negotiation, knowing the rudiments of effective strategy helps. But don't overestimate how quickly you'll learn. The art of negotiation is a complicated process that people have devoted their careers to studying, and since the early 1980s it has become a bona fide academic discipline.

The gurus of the field are Roger Fisher and William L. Ury of Harvard University, who wrote *Getting to Yes: Negotiating Agreement Without Giving In.* Their thesis, now widely accepted, is that most people think negotiation happens in one of two ways: fiercely or meekly. The hard bargainer sees negotiation as a contest of wills, issuing blustery demands backed up by threats. This "I win, you lose" school of dispute resolution tends to bring out inflexibility in the other side. Even if the parties reach agreement, the stage has been set for acrimony and possible retaliation. The other extreme is the "soft" style. The soft negotiator readily makes concessions to avoid conflict and is focused on developing a warm relationship, even at his or her own expense. The "you win, I lose" approach may lead to a signed contract, but the terms will be one-sided. Moreover, the other party might continue to expect such concessions.

Fisher and Ury advocate an alternative. "The method of principled negotiation," they write, "is to decide issues on their merits rather than through a haggling process focused on what each side says it will and will not do. It suggests that you look for mutual gains whenever possible, and that where your interests conflict, you should insist that the result be based on some fair standards independent of the will of the other side. The method of principled negotiation is hard on the merit, soft on the people. It employs no tricks and no posturing. Principled negotiation shows you how to obtain what you are entitled to and still be decent. It enables you to be fair while protecting you against those who would take advantage of your fairness."

Consultants and lawyers are referring to such negotiations when they talk about "win-win" agreements; the goal is to reach an accord that looks equally good to both sides. That is easier to do if you begin the process knowing precisely what you want as well as what you are willing to settle for. Once you've decided that, you will be in a good position to evaluate the final terms offered by the other side, a critical stage in the process. How does a doctor judge the merits of an offer? "The reason you negotiate is to produce something better than the results you can obtain without negotiating," write Fisher and Ury. "What are those results? What is that alternative? What is your BATNA—your Best Alternative to a Negotiated Agreement? *That* is the standard against which any proposed agreement should be measured. That is the only standard which can protect you both from accepting terms that are too unfavorable and from rejecting terms it would be in your interest to accept."

The best alternative for physicians who don't get the terms they want from one plan may be to negotiate with a competitor. On the other hand, if the first plan happens to be the best-run organization in the community and enrolls the largest employers, doctors may still profit from the contract. They would benefit from affiliation with an organization that is financially sound, ably administered, and capable of providing patients.

How sweet a deal doctors win depends, of course, on how much the managed-care plan needs them and how familiar they are with the types of concessions plans ordinarily make. Although the give-and-take of each negotiation is unique, the process has been played out so many times that patterns have emerged. Plans frequently strike the clause requiring physicians to indemnify the organization for all legal liability when patients sue. They often jettison the exclusivity clause as well, particularly for primary-care physicians. Obtaining adequate stop-loss reinsurance for protection against catastrophic medical expenses is rarely a stumbling block. Plans often agree to provide advance notice of substantial policy changes and to cap the amount a physician owes if the group's risk pool runs a deficit.

Physicians inexperienced in negotiating managed-care contracts may believe they have little else to gain. But those who have been through the process many times know they can achieve even more. A physician who agrees to accept the risk of capitation, for instance, might win a guarantee for a minimum volume of patients. Doctors treating all the patients they can handle may want the right to stop accepting new patients following 90 days' notice. Although managed-care organizations do not allow physicians to reject individual patients based on their medical needs, some grant doctors the right to close their doors to individuals who are disruptive or who routinely fail to appear for scheduled appointments. Doctors sometimes win a provision granting them a prorated share of the risk-pool surplus if they leave the plan before the contract expires. And it is always wise to request the right to renegotiate the contract before it automatically renews.

The biggest prize to win from an HMO goes to those who accept the greatest financial risk. Under the simplest form of capitation, a physician might receive $10 to $15 per patient per month to manage only the members' primary-care needs. Plans earmark an additional $70 or so for each member per month to cover the costs of specialists and hospitalization. Since most plans do not require physicians to cover deficits in those accounts, the primary-care doctor is typically at risk only for the base capitation.

The total amount, which covers all of a patient's medical needs, is a pie that can be divvied up in many different ways. The larger the slice that physicians cut for themselves, the more they can make—or lose. Solo practitioners and those in small groups generally prefer to settle for a bite-size piece, accepting a capitation rate that covers only primary care. Larger groups can afford to handle more risk and often opt for a much larger piece of the pie. Their capitation rate may approach $40 to $50 per patient per month because they are assuming financial responsibility for more comprehensive medical services.

"The marketplace is moving toward full-risk capitation," said Joel Shalowitz. In addition to running Northwestern's health services management program, Shalowitz cofounded a practice in 1983 that is growing at light speed. Since 1992 the group has doubled to include 10 internists and two affiliated pediatricians. They work at three sites in Chicago's northern suburbs, where about 15 percent of the population is enrolled in HMOs. Thanks to eight capitated HMO contracts and a slew of PPO contracts that Shalowitz hasn't even counted, the practice has added 200 new patients each month since 1992, and it gained 100 patients per month the preceding two years.

Unlike most physicians, who are new to the world of contract medicine, Shalowitz grew up with it. His father, also a physician, started an HMO with a network of multispecialty groups in the early 1970s. For a while father and son served as the HMO's medical director and associate medical director.

Shalowitz's business acumen and knowledge of the managed-care industry led him to pursue the stomach-churning realm of full-risk capitation. Half of the group's patients are covered by full-risk contracts, which generate about 70 percent of the practice's revenues.

Here's how the deal works. Shalowitz negotiates all the contracts for the group, which receives about $40 per patient per month for full-risk capitation. In exchange the internists provide all the usual primary care the HMO enrollees require. Unlike primary-care capitation, however, the full-risk approach requires the group to pay for all outpatient lab work and X-rays. More important, the practice is also financially responsible for the members' subspecialist needs. In other words, if one of Shalowitz's many Medicare patients who are enrolled in HMOs needs cataract surgery, the practice pays the cost. Furthermore, if a patient requires hospitalization, the group is responsible for the related costs to its primary-care physicians and for any specialists who may be called in—and no prior authorization is necessary. The only big-ticket items the group does not pay for are a hospital's charges for room and board and medications.

"Full-risk capitation turns the doctor into a mini-insurance company," Shalowitz said. "Insurance is a numbers game. Unless the plans bring you enough patients, there's no way you can adequately spread the risk." He figures his practice needs at least 200 patients from each plan to break even. If a practice is affiliated with a teaching hospital, it is likely to attract patients whose illnesses are more problematic than average; it would require as many as 400 patients from each plan to spread the risk. An individual physician would probably have a hard time getting that many patients from one plan, since HMOs like to distribute their members over a broad base of doctors. For that reason a solo practitioner would probably be foolhardy to tackle comprehensive capitation.

At first glance it might seem that one giant variable determines whether or not full-risk capitation turns out to be a good deal for a practice: the dollar amount of the capitation rate. Not so, said Shalowitz. That is the issue that managed-care plans are least likely to budge on. "There's not a tremendous amount of room for negotiation," he said. "All the plans in a given market pay within a few dollars of each other, since the capitation rate is a percentage of the gross premiums they charge. And most HMOs in any given area have fairly similar premiums." One provision a physician might want to bargain for, though, is an "escalator," which requires a capitation rate to rise in proportion to an HMO's gross premium rate. Unfortunately most escalators run in two directions: up and down. If a plan with an adjustable capitation rate lowers its premium rates—which sometimes happens in highly competitive markets—capitation rates go down as well.

If he is unable to haggle much over the capitation rate, how does Shalowitz turn a full-risk contract into a lucrative deal for his practice? First, he subcontracts all the specialty work on a competitive basis. "We look at quality and price," he said, "and it is truly in that order." Shalowitz added that he hasn't awarded any contracts to specialists merely because they charge lower fees than others. In fact, "all the physicians we've contracted with have been the same ones we use for our fee-for-service patients," he said.

The key that makes the full-risk contract pay off is the lower rates Shalowitz has won from specialists. He has far more incentive to negotiate hard for lower rates than the managed-care plans do "because it's our money," he said. For example, Medicare currently reimburses Chicago-area ophthalmologists $2,400 to perform cataract surgery; the total bill averages about $5,000. Shalowitz, however, negotiated a fee of $1,200 with his group's ophthalmologist, and the total cost for the procedure runs about $2,400. Assuming that the managed-care plans Shalowitz contracts with follow Medicare guidelines, which is likely, the money they calculate that his group needs for cataract procedures is twice as high as the group's actual expenses. The practice pockets the difference. Multiply the $2,600 savings by the number of cataract operations the group's patients require each year, and the dollars add up. Then imagine similar savings from each of the procedures specialists frequently perform, and you have the makings of a highly profitable enterprise.

As the popularity of full-risk capitation grows, more primary-care physicians are negotiating fees directly with specialists, who in turn are increasingly willing to accept lower fees in order to gain more patients. Another common development is that specialists are performing all the components of a procedure for a single negotiated rate. A man being tested for prostate cancer, for example, is usually sent to a hospital for an ultrasound test, which, if positive, might be followed by a needle-guided biopsy. Ordinarily Shalowitz's practice would receive separate bills from the radiologist who performed the ultrasound test, the urologist who did the biopsy, and the pathologist who examined the tissue, as well as bills from the facilities where the procedures were performed. The cost is high, and the bills are plentiful.

A urologist commonly used by Shalowitz's group offered to provide all the services in one package. "The urologist does everything himself," Shalowitz said. "He bought an ultrasound machine and does the test. He does the biopsy in his office instead of in the hospital. He brings the specimen down one floor to our office, and we send it out to the lab. The pathology analysis is just one item in our monthly lab bill. And the only other bill we pay is the one to the urologist." Specialists who offer packaged services for frequently performed procedures can market them either to capitated primary-care physicians or directly to managed-care organizations. This type of packaging is a creative way for besieged specialists to hold on to their threatened market shares.

A second way the group makes money on full-risk contracts is by knowing precisely what services a contract should cover and what should be excluded, or, in the parlance of capitation, "carved out." Managed-care plans routinely carve out treatment for mental illnesses and chemical dependency, for example, contracting with separate groups of physicians to handle those problems. Other procedures commonly excluded are reconstructive surgery, major joint replacements, neonatal complications, open-heart surgery, and other complex operations. Just about everything else is up for grabs. Should a capitation rate of about $40 include physical or occupational therapy? Should the group be financially responsible for durable medical equipment? Providing the right answer is critical. If a group agrees to cover too many of the wrong services, the costs could exceed the reimbursements. "There are a lot of different ways to cut this," Shalowitz said, "so you have to be very precise about what the capitation covers and what each component is worth." Groups that are large enough might want to hire an actuarial or accounting firm such as Arthur Andersen to make such evaluations.

The third way to make full-risk care profitable concerns the HMOs' hospital funds, which pay outpatient surgical-facility fees and most inpatient charges, except for the services of specialists, which the capitation rate covers. Each HMO Shalowitz contracts with sets aside a fund to cover hospital costs incurred by the practice. According to Shalowitz, a well-negotiated contract usually requires an HMO to give the practice half of any money remaining in the fund at the end of the contract year. "You can get some reasonable fees and good cash flow doing capitated care," said Shalowitz, "but the large profits are made by sharing in the plan's hospital fund."

A managed-care plan under the full-risk arrangement is not overly concerned with how long a patient remains hospitalized. It shifts the burden of making that call to the capitated physicians. Although it obviously pays for physicians to get their patients back home sooner rather than later, a premature release can be disastrous. "Ethics aside, it's a stupid business decision to release someone too early," Shalowitz said, since it can lead to to potentially expensive complications and malpractice charges.

On the other hand, if a physician can get a well patient discharged early, the group will profit. "Physicians can do a lot of creative things to get patients out of a hospital," said Shalowitz. For example, they could arrange for skilled nursing care, which is far less expensive than a day in the hospital. In the fee-for-service world, if healthy patients wanted to remain hospitalized an extra day because no one was able to pick them up or a spouse was out of town, their physicians wouldn't mind. They'd get paid for an extra bedside visit while also keeping the patient happy. In the capitated system, Shalowitz said, "the physician could pay for a limo to take the patient home and a round-the-clock nurse and still save money."

Negotiating full-risk contracts is tricky and not something an inexperienced physician should attempt without good advice, particularly from a health care lawyer who has expertise in this area. But as Shalowitz said, "what makes or breaks these contracts are not points of law—they're business principles."

CHAPTER *three*

FORMING A NETWORK

An allergist in private practice in Atlanta realizes his livelihood is threatened: a group of competitors has won exclusive contracts with several managed-care organizations. The doctor spends several months meeting with other allergists, consultants, and lawyers to plot a counterattack. A neurologist in Miami spends two years and thousands of dollars organizing his peers into a brigade of neurology providers strong enough to protect their turf as managed care roars through south Florida. Cardiologists working in 41 cities across the country band together to revolutionize the delivery of cardiac care—and to keep control over their destinies.

Physicians throughout the United States are grappling with the problem of how to reposition themselves in a marketplace increasingly dominated by managed-care organizations. For specialists, who constitute about 70 percent of the country's 600,000 physicians, the issue isn't merely maintaining or expanding market share; it's survival.

The ranks of specialists have been swelling since the 1930s due to the prospect of generous incomes and a stream of fee-for-service patients whose insurers picked up the tab. The result: a shortage of general practitioners and an overabundance of specialists. In 1993 fewer than 25 percent of graduating medical students expressed interest in becoming generalists, down from 50 percent in 1961, according to Dr. Marc L. Rivo, director of the Division of Medicine of the Department of Health and Human Services.

As long as society tolerated the spiraling cost of health care, the marketplace absorbed the oversupply of providers. But now that health care purchasers are focused on lowering costs, specialists are caught in a vise. Their ranks are growing as demand for their services shrinks. According to health care consultant David Vogel, specialists constituted 95 percent of the physicians in the typical fee-for-service multispecialty group practice of the 1970s and early 1980s. But in the 1990s, if more than half of a practice's patients are enrolled in managed-care plans, the percentage of specialists in the group usually drops to about 40 percent.

The squeeze comes from HMOs. A managed-care plan controls costs by prohibiting members from scheduling appointments directly with specialists. Unless patients require immediate hospitalization, they must first see one of the HMO's primary-care gatekeepers, who have a strong incentive to minimize referrals. The less specialists' services are used, the more the plan saves, and HMOs share those savings with their gatekeepers.

If only a small percentage of the population belonged to HMOs, specialists would not feel so threatened. But nearly 80 percent of the U.S. population will be insured by managed-care organizations by 2000. Specialists needn't wait that long to assess the damage of the diminishing demand for their services, however; it's already obvious. Only four of every 10 patients who schedule appointments with orthopedic surgeons, for example, are referrals; the rest are walk-ins. In areas dominated by managed care, orthopedic surgeons are losing up to 60 percent of their patients to the primary-care gatekeepers. Several orthopedic surgeons on the East Coast, where managed care is relatively uncommon, report incessant phone calls from California peers begging to join their practices.

Walk-ins are diminishing even in areas where HMOs have not become dominant. In the affluent Chicago suburbs that feed Dr. Joel Shalowitz's 10-physician practice, patients with minor ailments were accustomed to heading straight for a specialist. "This is a sophisticated, demanding population," said Shalowitz. "But patients are discovering that the primary-care doctor can handle lots of simple problems that they thought could only be handled by a specialist—and for a much lower cost." Despite treating several thousand Medicare patients, for example, Shalowitz's practice needs only one or two ophthalmologists for all his patients' eye-care needs.

Another unnerving development for specialists is that while the number of people enrolled in HMOs is steadily increasing, the number of HMOs is decreasing. The number peaked in 1987, when there were 662. Since then many plans have either folded or merged, and the number has dropped to 546. In *Physicians and Managed Care*, David Vogel states that the industry's consolidation will continue because employers are searching for the broadest range of services from the fewest plans. A single managed-care organization that offers a variety of insurance plans is ultimately an employer's most appealing choice.

As an HMO strengthens its hold on a local market, one way it flexes its muscle is by slashing specialists' fees. In cities where HMOs grant annual cost-of-living increases to primary-care gatekeepers, the plans are simultaneously cutting reimbursements for specialists by as much as 15 percent. But HMOs aren't the only force driving down specialists' incomes. In January 1992 the Health Care Financing Administration adopted a new pay scale for Medicare providers, the Resource-Based Relative-Value Scale (RB-RVS),which health plans across the country are copying. Its complicated formula determines the dollar value of more than 4,000 medical procedures based on factors such as a physician's time, mental effort and judgment, technical skill, stress, and practice expenses. Although the equation is complex, the result is simple: the pay scale intentionally raises the fees for procedures commonly used by generalists—taking a patient's history, for example—and lowers the fees for invasive procedures performed by specialists.

The double whammy of managed care and RB-RVS hasn't turned specialists into paupers, but the effects are nonetheless sobering. According to an annual survey by the Medical Group Management Association, the median compensation of family practitioners in 1992 rose by 7 percent, from $105,646 in 1991 to $112,585. During the same period plastic surgeons' income dropped by 8 percent, from $215,178 to $197,500, and anesthesiologists' income fell 4.3 percent, from $245,000 to $235,000.

Specialists are reacting to these pressures in various ways. Some view the situation as a temporary economic setback and are simply doing nothing—a dangerous approach in an industry undergoing fundamental change. Others have chosen the opposite extreme,

"As some men get drunk on alcohol,
so he gets drunk on science."
—Leo Tolstoy

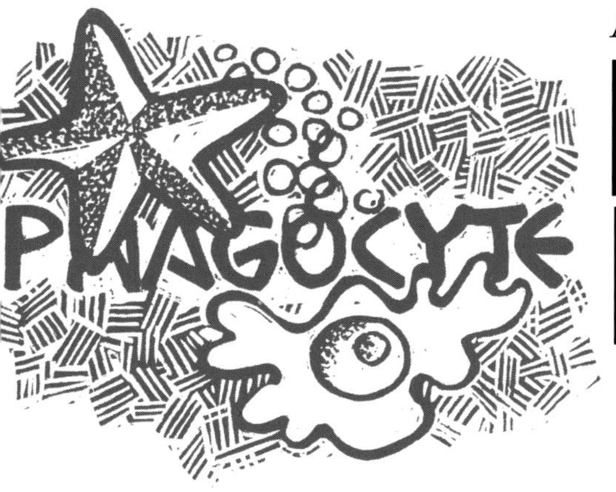

Miles is proud to present this series on...

Powerful Innovators

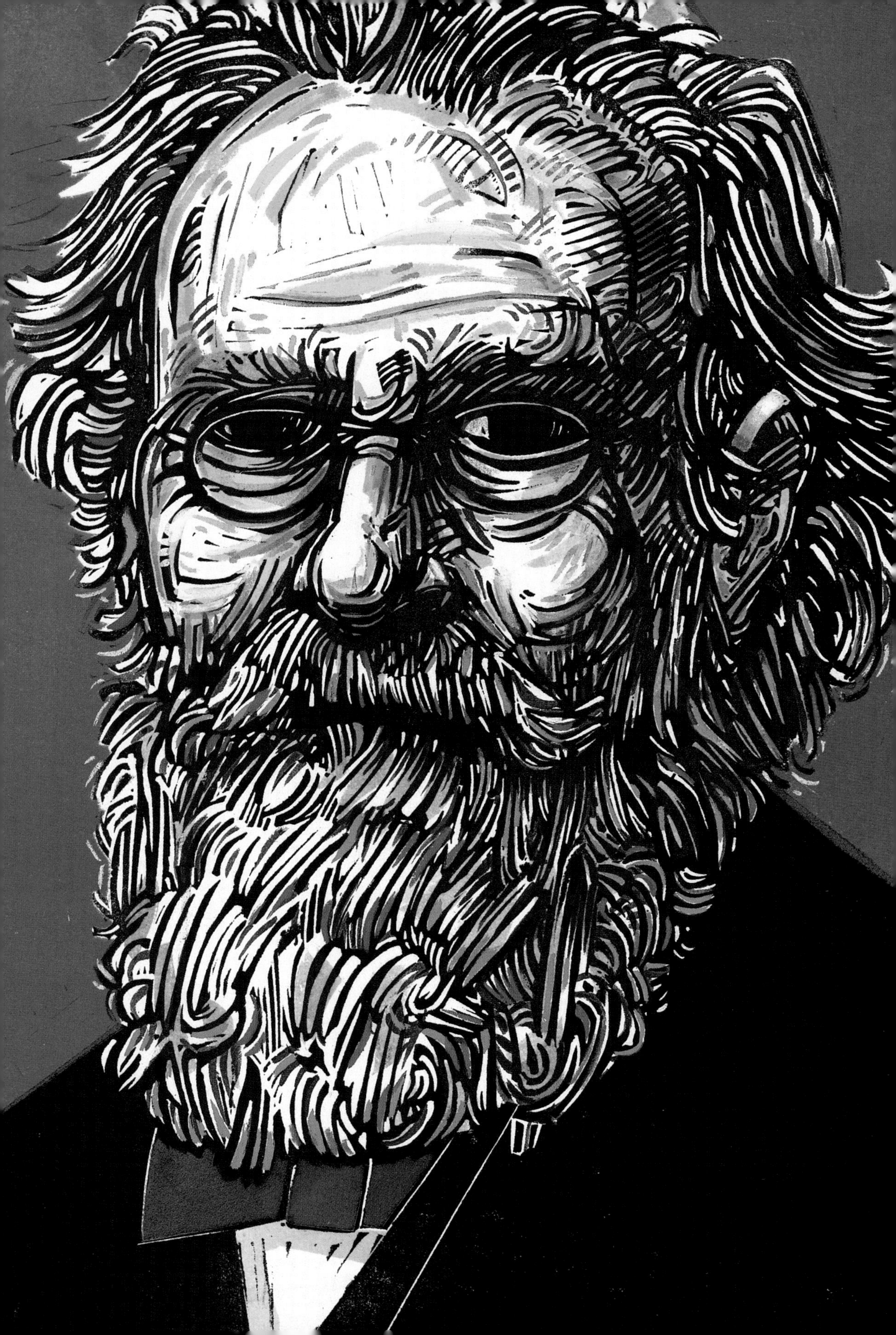

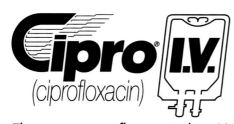

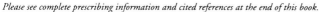

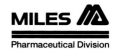

shucking their career paths and switching to primary-care practice.

Many practitioners conclude, however, that they can continue to be central to the system if they develop imaginative business strategies. Those who want to remain independent are marketing themselves to managed-care plans and their primary-care gatekeepers by cutting the costs of the procedures they perform frequently and by bundling the components of certain procedures into a single package.

For the majority of specialists, however, the smartest move is to join a single-specialty network. The chief advantage of networks is that physicians can negotiate collectively with health plans while remaining in their private practices. HMOs applaud the trend for several reasons: Networks save them the time and expense of obtaining specialists' services one provider at a time. They also allow HMOs to extend coverage to a wide area, a key feature to all purchasers of health care. In addition, a network of specialists can tailor its services to help an HMO save money in ways individual practitioners cannot. Finally, HMOs don't like to see their members go outside the plans for medical care, a problem that they curtail by contracting with a variety of single-specialty networks.

Acting collectively with competitors might seem to be a powerful weapon for specialists. What's to stop all the gastroenterologists in Oshkosh, for example, from forming a group and telling the town's HMOs: "If you want any stomach problems treated, you'll have to pay us what we want." That may sound like a pretty good plan for physicians who may feel puny compared to the behemoths of health care. But collective bargaining for fees is fraught with peril.

A group of Arizona physicians learned that lesson the hard way. In the late 1970s, 70 percent of the doctors in Maricopa County, fearing the impending arrival of managed-care plans, decided to make a preemptive strike. They formed a foundation whose purpose was to create a maximum reimbursement schedule, capping what the foundation could pay its members. To Maricopa County's physicians, the concept no doubt seemed a clever way to protect their incomes. To Arizona's attorney general, however, the scheme was a violation of the state's antitrust laws: competitors cannot as a group decide on fees, whether maximum or minimum, without affecting competition in the marketplace.

In 1982, after a series of legal setbacks, the doctors appealed their case to the U.S. Supreme Court. The Court came down on the defendants "like a ton of bricks," said Frances Miller, a professor specializing in health care law at the Boston University School of Law. The ruling states unequivocally that competing doctors cannot band together to set fees.

The Maricopa case instantly achieved landmark status; before the Supreme Court's ruling, federal antitrust laws had not been applied to the business activities of doctors. The Court's ruling forever changed the business of medicine by proclaiming that antitrust law "does not distinguish the medical profession from any other provider of goods and services."

Since then the Department of Justice and the Federal Trade Commission have examined physicians' joint ventures through a legal microscope. Doctors already reeling from federal regulations, insurance paperwork, and discounted fees have yet another nonclinical issue to worry about. In the 1990s a handbook on antitrust law may be almost as valuable to a doctor as the *Physicians' Desk Reference*. "The antitrust laws put physicians at great risk if they don't know what they're doing," said Miller. "Much of the action in antitrust law is now in health care."

Before entering into network arrangements, physicians should brush up on the basics of antitrust law. The price of ignorance is steep: violations are criminal offenses that carry maximum penalties for individual physicians of three years in prison and $350,000 in fines. Incorporated practices could be fined as much as $10 million. Doctors convicted on separate civil charges, which could be filed by a competitor, a patient, or a third-party payer, could find themselves paying treble damages plus picking up the tab for all attorneys' fees. If a judge determined that the damage of the physicians' anticompetitive action was $100,000, for example, the court would assess a penalty of $300,000.

The rules governing antitrust are fairly straightforward. The first and most basic statute is the Sherman Act, enacted in 1890 to promote free enterprise. A fundamental principle of federal antitrust laws is that they protect competition, not competitors. Those laws may be violated whenever the process of competition in a particular market is harmed.

The worst types of antitrust offenses physicians can commit boil down to a few sentences: If competing physicians in a community agree about what fees to charge for certain services, they are guilty of price-fixing. If they decide as a group to refuse to deal with a managed-care plan unless it agrees to their terms, they are guilty of a group boycott. If they decide to divide the market by having one group serve the north side of town while the other group sticks to the south side, they are guilty of a market-allocation arrangement.

Courts regard these infringements as so threatening to the free flow of commerce that they are treated as per se offenses—legalese for antitrust crimes always considered anticompetitive regardless of their measurable effect on a market. If you commit one of those crimes and get caught, you're in a heap of trouble. Authorities don't even need a smoking gun to win convictions; they don't have to uncover a formal contract or notes scribbled on a cocktail napkin. All it takes is a group of competitors who meet, agree to stifle competition in a particular way, and then execute their plan.

Collusion is the basis of the offense. Individual physicians can shun any health plan they please and not worry about a charge of boycotting. The courts view members of a fully integrated practice as single players in an antitrust sense, so they can freely discuss fees without fear of price-fixing charges. And joint ventures, which involve partial integration of physicians' practices, fall under the more lenient rule of reason rather than the per se rule. In other words, in this gray area of antitrust law, the courts do not automatically view pricing arrangements as restraints of trade; instead they rely on evidence to determine whether the venture has hurt consumers.

Facing such formidable legal obstacles, how can a group of competing doctors band together without violating the law? Because this question was on the minds of so many physicians, federal antitrust enforcement agencies issued a policy statement in September 1993 to clarify the rules and establish antitrust "safety zones." The document states that the government "will not challenge a physician network joint venture comprised of 20 percent or less of the physicians in each physician specialty . . . who practice in the relevant geographic area and share substantial financial risk." Although the definition of "relevant geographic area" remains fuzzy and requires a lawyer's interpretation in each case, in general the area is defined as a city or county. "Substantial financial risk" is not well defined either, but the document does offer two examples: capitation and financial incentives such as withhold agreements. Again, a lawyer can help doctors determine whether they meet the criteria.

If a network fails to meet these criteria, it has not necessarily broken the law. But the authorities might challenge it using the rule of reason, a potentially time-consuming and expensive process. Basically the government wants to make sure the network is not a sham, an outfit whose only purpose is to fix prices, like the one set up by the physicians in Maricopa County. Networks will get a green light to proceed if they can demonstrate that the participants are indeed sharing substantial financial risks or if they are creating a low-cost, high-quality service for consumers that offsets any effect they have on competition.

Forming a network can be a valuable strategy for specialists who want greater access to managed-care patients—if they are attentive to the legalities. "It's the best of both worlds," said Dr. Stan M. Fineman, an allergist in Atlanta. "Those of us in the network keep our own practices, so we maintain our autonomy—and we're able to maintain our patient base."

With ample supplies of both people and pollen, Southern cities are attractive places for allergists to set up shop. Under the fee-for-service system, Fineman's solo practice thrived. But in 1989, when some managed-care plans arrived in town, he faced the most difficult challenge of his career. The plans studied Atlanta's supply of allergists and saw that most were in private practice like Fineman or in two-person groups. But one group of 12 allergists operated out of several offices scattered around the metropolitan area. For the HMOs, deciding which allergists to add to their panel of providers was a no-brainer. Why spend the time and money identifying a dozen good individual allergists in the right geographic areas, then negotiate a contract with each one, when it was possible to get everything they wanted by dealing with a single large group?

Although Fineman was prepared for rough times once managed care hit Atlanta, he was caught off guard by what happened next. Some of the city's HMOs awarded exclusive capitated contracts to the 12-doctor group, cutting off all other allergists from those HMOs. Suddenly denied access to a large population of potential customers, Fineman realized that he had to act quickly to save his practice. He based his strategy on two premises: he wanted to remain a solo practitioner, and he wanted to compete head-to-head with larger practices for managed-care contracts.

The only way to achieve his goal, he decided, was to create a single-specialty network. Although his medical training did not include courses in designing and implementing innovative business plans, he was determined to fight. He spent several months meeting with the city's other solo allergists, certain they must feel as besieged as he did. As he explained the dangerous effect managed care posed to those who remained independent, his colleagues listened eagerly. Although not everyone saw the wisdom of his strategy, "it was not that hard to get people on board," Fineman recalled.

He won the tacit support of enough of his peers to be a force in Atlanta's allergy market. What he lacked, however, was the legal and administrative expertise to formalize the group. After making a few inquiries, he selected Gates, Moore & Company, a national health care consulting firm in Atlanta, to help him get the network started.

The first step was the selection of doctors to include in the network. It's not unlike throwing a party: invite everyone in the neighborhood and you will inevitably attract some ne'er-do-wells. Since HMOs prefer providers who are board-certified, work in the areas where the HMO members live, have privileges with major hospitals, and are known to be clinically adept, the network's organizers used those criteria to select its 15 members.

The group organized itself as a taxable not-for-profit corporation. The structure is called a messenger-model network, the most common format used by specialists who collectively contract with managed-care plans. Its method of operation is fairly simple: The consultants manage the corporation's business affairs and negotiate capitated contracts with HMOs on behalf of the network's allergists. They take 5 percent of the HMOs' monthly payments to run the network. Each month the physicians submit claims itemizing their work, and the network managers reimburse them according to a set fee schedule.

This arrangement sidesteps the most treacherous antitrust pitfalls. First, the network's members are sharing substantial financial risk by working under a capitated payment system. Second, the physicians avoid charges of price-fixing because they are not collectively negotiating the price of their services. The network manager, playing the role of "messenger," does it for them. The messenger develops a fee proposal and submits it to the physicians for approval. The allergists continue to set their own fees for their non-HMO patients; antitrust laws prohibit the group members from discussing their private fee schedules with one another.

Joining a network may provide doctors with a way to bargain collectively, but it hardly guarantees a financial windfall. Capitation is a lot trickier for specialists than it is for generalists. Primary-care physicians receive $10 to $15 a month for each of their HMO patients. Since most HMOs allow their members to schedule appointments with primary-care doctors only, those doctors can receive a flood of patients—and dollars.

For specialists the arrangement is significantly different. HMOs prefer to contract with one network per specialty, making it responsible for treating all of a plan's members. The capitation rate varies according to the specialty and location of the practice. Depending on the market, HMOs pay allergy networks a capitation rate of 30 to 60 cents per month multiplied by the number of people enrolled in the HMO, regardless of how many members see an allergist. In Atlanta the going rate is about 50 cents. If an allergy network contracts with an HMO that has 30,000 members, the monthly check would total $15,000. While the HMO's capitation rate stays firm at 50 cents, the number of plan members, and hence the plan's payment to the network, fluctuates each month.

Although most HMOs don't experience wild swings in membership from month to month, it does happen. It's not uncommon, for example, for an employer to leave one plan for another. If the arrangement seems a little like playing the stock market, that's because it is. The best you can do is bet on a blue chip, but as any shareholder of IBM knows, even the mighty can tumble.

Merely affiliating with an HMO is more difficult for specialists than for primary-care doctors. A general practitioner can window-shop, checking out all the HMOs in town to see which offer the highest capitation rates and best incentive programs, and then choose the most attractive ones. Specialist networks, on the other hand, are required to submit bids. If two or three networks of allergists submit bids to the same HMO, it evaluates the competing offers and chooses one.

Although a network's administrative manager prepares the bid, physicians should understand its basic components, which reflect how the network will function. A network markets itself to health plans principally through the bid material. Computing a dollar amount that's competitive yet adequate is a priority. To do a proper job, the manager needs enough data to estimate how many people per thousand are likely to visit an allergist each year, what treatments they need most frequently, what cases cost the most, and what ailments are the most difficult to treat. Setting fees has traditionally been somewhat arbitrary, but not in the fiercely competitive marketplace of the 1990s. Doctors are finally applying the hard business principles of cost accounting to medical services, said L. Michael Fleischman, the partner at Gates, Moore & Company who manages Fineman's network of allergists. "When Maxwell House decides to charge a certain amount for a pound of coffee, the price reflects the costs of transportation, advertising, labor, and so on," said Fleischman. "Doctors have never done that—until now."

How does cost accounting work in an allergist's practice? "It's a difficult process," said Fineman, "but we're trying to figure out how much it really costs us, for example, to do an allergy evaluation for a patient. A normal charge might be $200, but it probably doesn't cost us that much in terms of time and material. It may not even cost us $100; it may cost only $75. But if we can get $100 for it, we're still making some money—not much, but we're making a profit."

Managed-care plans don't automatically award a contract to the network that comes in with the lowest bid. A properly prepared bid also makes a case for the network's clinical and managerial superiority. But such claims are meaningless unless they can be documented; a network needs methods to ensure that its physicians are delivering high-quality care and are not performing unnecessary procedures. The way Fineman's network handles these issues is typical: At the top of the organization is a three-physician executive committee responsible for checking the credentials of new network members and dropping those who don't measure up. Another committee handles peer review, investigating complaints by patients or by an HMO's medical director. A third, the quality-assurance committee, establishes clinical protocols and conducts spot checks of colleagues' charts to make sure no one is performing more tests than patients require.

To an HMO these committees indicate a network's commitment to the principles of managed care. If the committee members do their jobs well, the network manager will include the minutes of their meetings as part of the bid, along with data showing how the group treats its patients. These are hardly ancillary documents. "They are essential tools that demonstrate a network's strength," said Fleischman.

A surefire way for a network to endear itself to an HMO is to help the plan control a cost that has gotten out of hand. A savvy network of urologists, for example, might ask an HMO to identify the five or so urology conditions that cost the HMO the most in hospitalization expenses each year. The urologists would then propose a deal to the HMO: "At the end of a year, give us 25 cents of every dollar we save you through our treatment of those five conditions." Many HMOs are more than happy to agree to such arrangements.

A few years ago Fineman's network profited from that kind of deal. An HMO the group contracted with said that one of its highest costs resulted from the hospitalization of asthmatics, particularly children. The allergists and the HMO decided that if the specialists cut down the number of asthma patients who required hospitalization by a certain amount, the specialists would get 10 percent of the savings. They volunteered considerable time teaching the HMO's primary-care physicians how to manage the care of pediatric asthmatics and educating the parents as well. At the end of a year, the allergists had saved the HMO $300,000 in asthma-related hospital expenses.

For Fineman creating the network was an inspired idea. "My practice definitely would have suffered if I hadn't gone this route," he said. As for the allergists who ignored him back in 1989, well, they're out of luck. "Some have come back asking to join," said Fineman. "But if they work in an area where we already have a member, there's no advantage for us to include them. We don't need them."

The initiative to form a network usually comes from independent physicians who feel threatened by larger groups and see safety in numbers. But a growing number of insurance companies are also creating such arrangements; they want to maintain good relations with providers while shifting the cost of processing claims.

In 1991 a large insurance company asked Dr. Richard P. Singer to form a single-specialty network of neurologists who would provide care exclusively for the health plan's members in a three-county area in southern Florida. At the time Singer headed a private practice that included three other neurologists who worked out of three offices in Dade and Broward counties.

Even though the Miami area has been a hotbed of managed care, most specialists have chosen to avoid it. Not Singer. The 46-year-old neurologist started treating managed-care patients in 1982 and says his practice was one of the first groups of private board-certified neurologists in south Florida that agreed to see HMO patients. "We depend on referrals," he explained. "It's not of great import to us whether the referrals come from a private doctor or an HMO doctor."

His practice style caught the eye of one of his major insurers, which asked him to establish the network. As someone who wanted to stay ahead of managed care, Singer accepted the challenge. The resulting business plan was ambitious and groundbreaking.

For the concept to work, Singer had to undertake two formidable tasks. The first involved identifying enough highly regarded board-certified neurologists to cover the several hundred miles of territory served by the insurance company. It was not an easy assignment, Singer said, because many of the obvious candidates had had bad experiences with HMOs. Some complained of reimbursement delays. Others angrily recounted tales of payment denials. Many of the neurologists Singer approached dealt with the insurer he was representing, but not with its managed-care division. Some preferred to keep it that way.

Executing the other part of the plan was even more difficult. The insurance company didn't want to absorb the high expense of receiving, reviewing, and processing the network's claims for medical services. In fact, from the insurance company's perspective, the highlight of the network idea was to save lots of money by placing that costly burden on someone else's shoulders. To Singer, accepting that responsibility seemed a worthwhile gamble.

Singer and a partner spent two years and many thousands of dollars creating a management company to run the network. They formed a for-profit entity and hope to recoup their investment through management fees. One major problem was finding liability insurance in case someone sued one of the network's physicians. "We couldn't find a company that had ever underwritten a management company," Singer said, "but we couldn't proceed without insurance because south Florida is one of the most litigious areas of the country." Another tough hurdle was finding a computer company to write the software programs for processing the claims. The partners stuck with it, and Singer became both a practicing neurologist and the network director of Neurology Management Inc.

Here's how the system works: The management company negotiates a capitated contract with the insurance company and receives a certain fee per member per month based on the number of people enrolled in the HMO. The management company has a separate contract with the network neurologists; their reimbursements are tied to a modified fee-for-service schedule based on a relative-value-unit system similar to Medicare's RB-RVS. Most networks reimburse specialists in this fashion; it eliminates the price distortions and annual increases associated with the traditional usual-and-customary fee system.

The management company's chief task is to review, process, and pay the claims submitted by members. Clerical workers answer phones and handle the mail, but Singer assigned the job of reviewing the physicians' claims to a staff of two neurologists, a key feature that swayed reluctant physicians to join the network. "Their claims are being reviewed by their peers, not by a clerk in an insurance office 2,000 miles away," said Singer. "And the claims are paid within 10 days after the physicians submit their monthly bills."

A cynic might think such an approach invites danger, a fraternal spirit that encourages doctors to approve whatever bills their colleagues submit. Not so, said Singer. The management company has peer-review and quality-assurance committees just as Fineman's allergy network does. And capitation discourages doctors from performing unnecessary procedures. "The amount you get paid isn't a constant figure each month," Singer explained. "It depends on the total utilization within the network for the month. So by discouraging the use of, say, electrical nerve testing, there's more money to distribute for cognitive work. And that's the key to a successful network: understanding that the other doctors will get less in a particular month if there's overutilization." The network denies payment to member doctors for tests deemed unwarranted. "It happened more at the beginning," said Singer. "But once doctors caught on that they wouldn't be reimbursed, that behavior changed."

The prospect of receiving payments quickly, having claims reviewed by peers, and gaining access to a high volume of patients proved a tempting combination. At last count, 70 neurologists representing 20 practices belonged to the network.

Asked if he thinks the project has been worth the trouble, Singer replied, "If a lot of people sign up for managed care and doctors can't get access to them, they're going to end up feeling like Custer."

The beauty of the network concept is its elasticity. Networks are limited only by antitrust laws, market conditions, and their creators' imaginations. The majority are designed to serve metropolitan areas, and an increasing number cover hundreds of square miles. The country's most progressive single-specialty network is the National Cardiovascular Network, which includes doctors in 41 cities who have teamed up to provide high-quality cardiac care at substantial savings.

The network is made up of units consisting of a cardiology practice, a cardiovascular surgeon, and a hospital, said David M. Zacks, an Atlanta attorney who began creating the network in 1992 with Dr. William D. Knopf, a cardiologist. The network offers bypass surgery, angioplasty, cardiac catheterization, and other heart treatments to patients in 23 states. It offers its services to large companies and insurers at what's called a global capitation rate—a fixed fee that covers surgery, hospitalization, and every other expense associated with a particular procedure. The specialists, surgeons, and hospitals work out a formula to divide the revenue.

By sending clients a single, all-inclusive bill and by pooling expertise to standardize approaches to complicated heart procedures, the network's physicians hope to cut the cost of a typical $60,000 bypass operation by about 40 percent." We want to ensure that the customer gets value," said Zacks. "And value is defined as cost effectiveness plus high-quality outcomes. Our clients will get a bang for their buck if we can show that they can have quality while spending one less day in the hospital—that way, everybody wins."

To sell such a radical concept, Zacks and Knopf realized they had to limit membership to physicians who met demanding criteria. "Volume was essential," said Zacks. "You don't want someone who does just a few of these procedures each year. They get rusty." A cardiology practice doesn't get an invitation to join this club unless it performs a minimum of 500 bypass operations and 300 angioplasty procedures per year. If the threshold seems high, that's the idea. No one facing open-heart surgery wants an inexperienced surgeon. The network's doctors already perform about 15 percent of all heart-bypass operations and angioplasty procedures in the U.S. The physicians must also meet certain standards regarding rates of morbidity, mortality, complications, and readmissions, said Zacks

While Knopf worked out the complicated medical criteria, Zacks mapped out an equally sophisticated legal strategy. In the fall of 1993 the Department of Justice created a unit to review the proposed business plans of newly formed medical networks and decide whether they met antitrust guidelines. The unit was not exactly deluged with mail. Most network managers figured you had to be crazy to provide information to the government, that drawing attention to yourself could only lead to trouble, and that the government would spend an agonizingly long time reaching a decision.

But Zacks saw the possibility of prior government approval as an opportunity and wasted no time shipping the network's plan to the government. "This is a project of great magnitude," he explained. "Why go to the trouble and expense of putting it together if the Justice Department feels it is inappropriate? And if we know from the start that we're doing it right, why not let the doctors we want know that up front?"

The risk paid off. In November 1993 the Department of Justice issued its first letter of approval concerning physician joint ventures to the National Cardiovascular Network. As Zacks predicted, federal approval helped persuade the best doctors to sign up.

Could the same arrangement be applied to other complicated and costly medical procedures? "Unfortunately, there are no cookie-cutter approaches to medicine," said Zacks. But as he and others have proved, if specialists understand the market demands in their area, study the needs of the health plans and their primary-care physicians, and examine the advantages of forming a single- or multispecialty network, they may just spin the dross of managed care into gold.

CHAPTER *four*

The Versatile Merger

When managed-care plans and businesses hand out contracts, they look for medical practices that can do three things: treat more patients, accept more economic risk, and offer more services than the doctor next door. Consequently doctors in solo practice or in small groups face the gut-wrenching choice of giving up their autonomy or watching their incomes shrivel. A handful are retiring early, but the rest are scurrying for cover, searching for advice on how to affiliate with larger groups that have the market strength to survive in an increasingly rigorous environment.

The solution, they're told, is to "integrate," the health care buzzword of the 1990s. A chorus of lawyers, consultants, and trade publications sing the praises of horizontally integrated provider relationships and vertically integrated health delivery systems, then charge hefty fees to explain what all the high-class labels mean. They pull out schematic drawings showing a web of lines connecting physicians to newly invented corporate entities, which in turn are connected to hospitals, insurance companies, clinics, and patients.

Many doctors who practice in the handful of places where HMOs have existed for several decades favor such byzantine business arrangements. They long ago gave up private practice and formed groups that often include hundreds of practitioners. And they've created sophisticated ways of marketing themselves, involving unusual partnerships with hospitals and health plans.

But for the great majority of U.S. doctors, who live in places where managed care is just surfacing, integration is a foreign concept. In most communities clinics without walls, physician-hospital organizations, and hospital-affiliated management-service organizations simply don't exist. And even if they do crop up, they are not necessarily appropriate for everybody. Leaping from a fee-for-service private practice to a physician-hospital joint venture is like surfacing too quickly from the ocean floor. You may get the bends. How, then, can physicians position themselves to at least maintain their market share regardless of where they live? Is there anything they can do short of plunging into a vertically integrated something or other?

For most physicians, the answer is as simple—and as complicated—as merging with other groups. The merger of two or more practices may seem like a mundane strategic maneuver compared with the flashier designs the experts tout, but it has the appeal of practicality. For everyone from internists in Indianapolis to orthopedists in Oswego, merging with other groups is a readily available and relatively painless way to become a more attractive competitor in the managed-care marketplace. In the wardrobe of strategic options, the merger is like a blazer: it may not turn heads, but its versatility can't be matched, and it will never go out of style.

Although mergers, like networks, are governed by federal antitrust laws, the rules are not overly burdensome. The Clayton Antitrust Act prohibits mergers that may "substantially lessen competition or tend to create a monopoly." Mergers involving noncompetitors—an orthopedic and a neurology group, for instance—do not worry authorities. But mergers involving competitors, such as two orthopedic groups, may attract unwelcome attention from enforcement agencies because the groups could use their newly acquired power to raise the cost of care in their communities. A rule of thumb is that problems can arise when the combined groups represent more than 35 percent of the specialists in their market. Even then the move is not necessarily illegal, but it could raise eyebrows. If the government decides that a merger has harmed competition, it can force the group apart.

From a business standpoint, mergers are a smart move. Most physicians never see 55 to 65 percent of what they collect; that's how much is typically eaten up by rent or mortgage payments, personnel, equipment, supplies, malpractice insurance, and other overhead expenses.

When two parties merge, overhead may or may not decline, but gross revenues should increase. Furthermore the cost of running a practice usually decreases, because a group of 10 or so can take advantage of economies of scale. Say two obstetricians, two gynecologists, and three pediatricians merge. Instead of each practice paying rent for separate office space, the group settles into one facility and saves thousands of dollars annually. Instead of each practice paying salaries and benefits to five employees, the combined group requires a support staff of perhaps only 10, saving thousands more. Instead of each doctor paying retail prices for supplies, the new group orders in bulk, paying wholesale and slicing even more off the bottom line. Add the savings from group insurance policies and you have the makings of a lean, cost-efficient, and profitable enterprise—the goal of every business.

As a result of these economies of scale, the new seven-physician group could soon have increased working capital—a luxury that high overhead usually precludes. These surplus funds can pay for a remodeled office with additional exam rooms, a new computer system to expedite billings and collections, the latest ultrasound unit, or whatever else a thriving practice requires to stay one step ahead of competitors. Since most doctors don't have the time—or the inclination—to handle management details, their shrewdest investment might be to hire an experienced administrator to oversee the group's business affairs and to negotiate managed-care contracts.

The bright economic picture that results from a well-planned merger makes it superior to a network. Belonging to a network is like going on a date: independent physicians approach HMOs arm-in-arm, then return to their respective offices, each a self-contained cost center. They might expand their patient loads, but their overheads remain unchanged. After a few years, once the network's members know one another's personal and clinical styles, they sometimes propose a more serious business relationship: the marriage of their practices.

Moreover, group practices can frequently market themselves more effectively than networks. A network of allergists, for example, treats only people with allergy problems and must compete with the area's other specialists in the field. A group practice that includes obstetricians, gynecologists, and pediatricians, on the other hand, provides medical care for a much larger population; in addition, doctors can deliberately design a group to be the only three-specialty practice in a community. For those reasons, a well-balanced primary-care group—assuming its physicians are clinically adept and cost-conscious—will easily attract contracts from businesses and health plans.

If the benefits of merging practices are so obvious, why isn't everyone merging? Well, for the same reason every adult isn't married. Some lucky souls find the right mate before they even know they are looking, some search for years before they find the perfect partner, and others want nothing other than their independence. Similarly, just as some couples marry prematurely, some physicians plunge into a merger before they've become fully acquainted with their new partners. Both scenarios are likely to end in divorce.

The most important ingredient in a prospective merger is harmony. No matter how strategically sound it may be, the merger of two or more practices is doomed if the physicians don't get along. "Physicians routinely talk about the theory of merger," said attorney Alice Gosfield, "but a lot back off when they see what's involved."

What's involved, more often than not, is an acute case of ambivalence. Many doctors know they should realign themselves with peers, but they are accustomed to doing things their own way; accommodation is not their strong suit. Gosfield recalls a visit in 1993 from three small physician groups that wanted to merge. A lack of resolve surfaced immediately. Rather than merge straight away, the doctors wanted to do so incrementally. They proposed remaining in separate offices and uniting only their billing and collection activities. Gosfield explained that the antitrust laws prohibit economic competitors from merging their billing operations. You can't do it halfway, Gosfield told them, so let's talk about what merging really means.

When she told them that they would have to split the overhead, one doctor asked, "You mean the cost of things like furniture and employees?" Gosfield nodded. "Just a minute," another physician said. "His patients sit on plastic chairs. He pays his staff $11,000 a year. They can't spell or type." "Well," the accused physician replied, "I've been in your waiting room, with those damn Audubon prints all over the walls. Your patients sit on Queen Anne chairs, and you pay your girls $35,000 a year. We'd all go broke." Needless to say, they never merged.

"For a merger to be successful," Gosfield said, "the participating physicians must have common practice values, and they must be capable of compromise."

"As long as I have a water tap, a flame, and some blotting paper, I can just as well work in a barn."

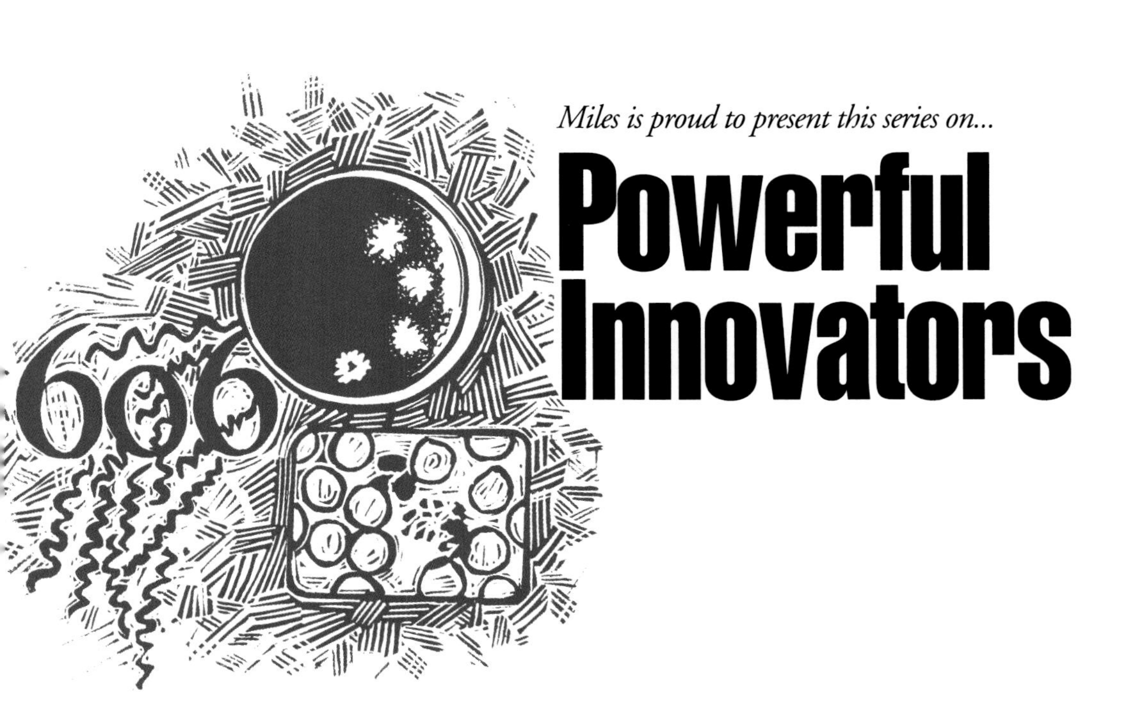

Miles is proud to present this series on...

Powerful Innovators

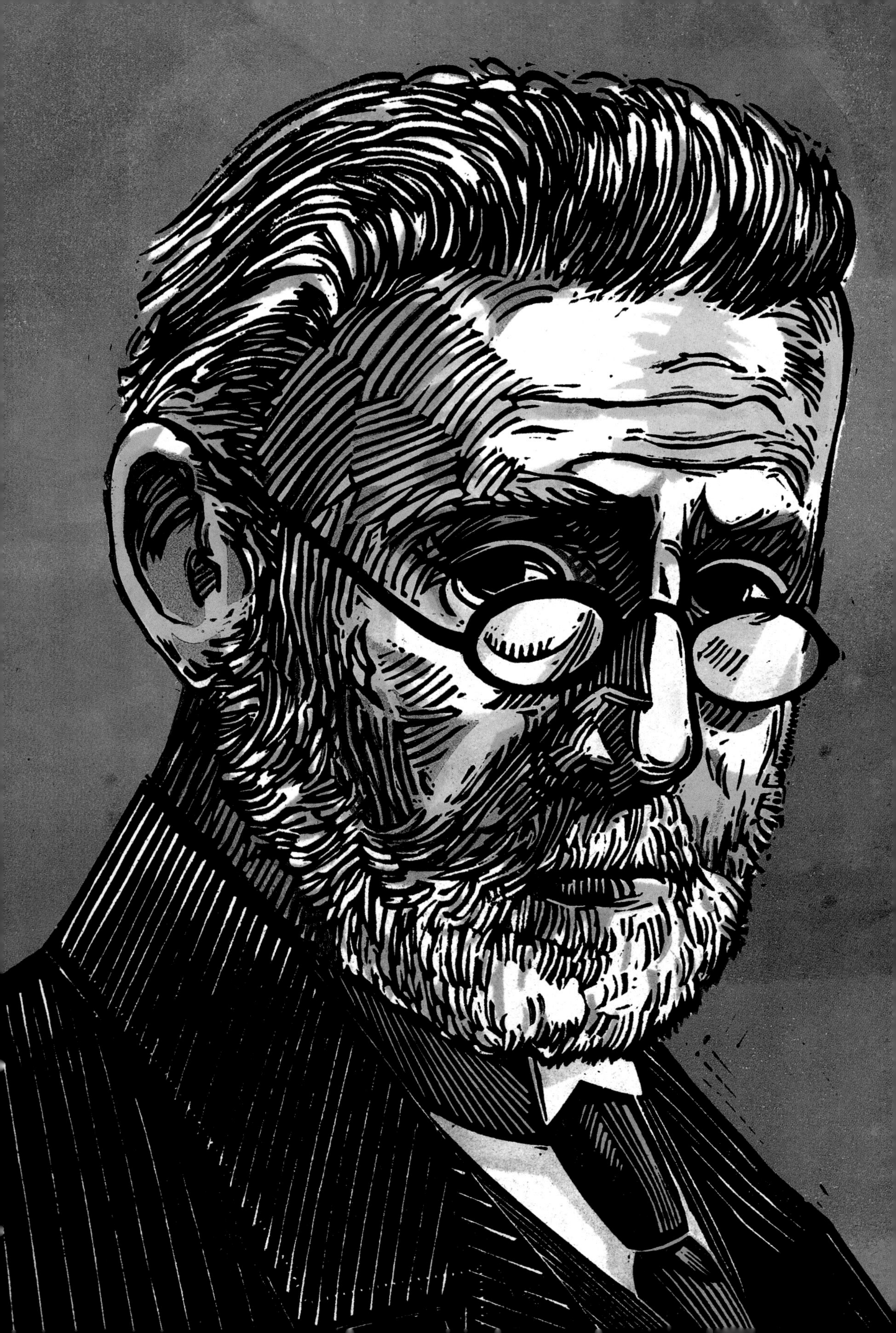

Powerful Physician

Paul Ehrlich (1854-1915)

Even as a child, Ehrlich displayed the curiosity and imagination we associate with brilliant scientists. His vivid descriptions earned him the nickname "Dr. Fantasy."

Ehrlich proved a gifted, intuitive experimenter who astonished his colleagues with the accuracy of his work.

In 1908, Ehrlich was awarded a share of the Nobel Prize in medicine and physiology for his research on immunity and serum. He spent the better part of two decades studying chemicals to find those that would selectively kill bacteria without harming humans. Interestingly, his most famous discovery came after he won the Nobel Prize, when he identified a compound known as "606"—naming it Salvasan (from salvation)—and identified its usefulness against syphilis—one of the most feared, albeit least discussed, diseases at that time.

Ehrlich's work marked the beginning of modern chemotherapy. Many believe that he set in motion the quick discovery of cures for many infectious diseases.

Powerful Antimicrobial

Today, in lower respiratory infections, some pathogens are no longer routinely susceptible to traditional agents. One important reason the power of Cipro® stands out is its unique mode of action. It allows the power of Cipro® to remain unaffected by ß-lactamase or plasmid-mediated resistance. And cross-resistance, which often limits the usefulness of other classes of antibiotics, is not a problem reported with Cipro®. In fact, Cipro® kills susceptible pathogens* during all four phases of cell growth.†*

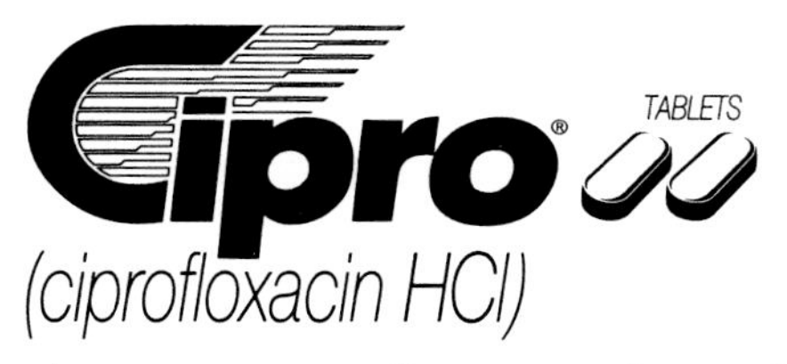

The most potent fluoroquinolone.[1-3‡]

*Due to susceptible strains of indicated pathogens. See indicated organisms in prescribing information.
†Data on file, Miles Inc Pharmaceutical Division.
‡*In vitro* activity does not necessarily imply a correlation with *in vivo* results.

See full prescribing information at the end of this book.

If the participating doctors are compatible and they have a strategic reason for aligning, the mechanics should not derail the process. Usually the new group organizes itself as a for-profit professional corporation, which means in most states that only physicians can be shareholders; in other words, the group cannot raise capital by selling shares to the public. If the new group contains 35 or fewer shareholders, it can opt for "S corporation" status. Corporations adhering to that subchapter of the Internal Revenue Code pass their income along to their physician shareholders, who report it on their personal tax returns and pay individual rather than corporate rates. For several years prior to 1993, when individual rates topped out at 31 percent and corporate rates were in the high 30s, an S corporation made a lot of sense. But in 1993 individual rates exceeded corporate ones, so physicians considering such a move should consult a tax expert.

Many doctors mistakenly believe that in a professional corporation their assets are protected if someone in the group is sued. In fact state laws determine whether a physician's legal shield is made of tinfoil or titanium. In some states physician shareholders are vulnerable only if the corporation is sued for nonmedical reasons. In other jurisdictions, if a physician loses a malpractice suit and the judgment exceeds his or her insurance coverage, the doctors in the corporation foot the bill. Several states limit the doctors' legal liability.

A merger involving seven or eight primary-care doctors is the equivalent of forming a multimillion-dollar-a-year business. Those who appreciate the gravity of the undertaking will map out a plan for governance. Without it dissension can escalate, fiscal issues fester, and a multimillion-dollar company fail.

There is no inherently right or wrong way to govern a newly merged group. All that matters is that the doctors agree before the merger to a system for making group decisions. Some groups boast of their ability to reach unanimous agreement. The larger the group, however, the more difficult unanimity becomes. Further complicating an egalitarian approach, as the often-heard truism puts it, is that managing a group of physicians is like trying to herd cats.

Doctors can simplify the governing process by adopting a few organizational measures. According to most experts, the first step is to create an executive committee composed of one doctor from each practice. The board should meet once every two weeks or so to discuss matters such as selecting a new computer system or hiring a new broker to beef up the pension plan. All of the group's doctors should get together at least quarterly to vote on such issues as hiring additional physicians and making major purchases.

Agreement among converging groups is most elusive when the talk turns to money. Up-front cash payments are not required when groups merge since they are merely combining assets. First an accountant figures out the accounts receivable and the total of each group's hard assets, such as equipment and real estate. If the assets are equivalent, there's no problem. But if one of the groups has amassed considerable debt, the others cannot be expected to shoulder someone else's burden. Doctors can generally work out such discrepancies without too much fuss. If group A has a $50,000 debt and the other practices are debt-free, then the group A doctors simply receive less compensation than the others until they have reached economic parity.

The most difficult issue is figuring out how to distribute income. The main reason specialists rarely merge with general practitioners is that they represent opposite poles of the medical world, and the differences are most visible in their paychecks. How does a group equitably distribute money brought in by surgeons and family practitioners? Should they share overhead equally? Should they retain the same percentage of their collections? Should productivity determine compensation? Should the physicians place their incomes into a common pot and divide it equally? Try floating that idea to a group of surgeons and they wouldn't know whether to scream or laugh. The most common compromise is to divide half the revenue equally and distribute the other half according to productivity.

Finding ways to distribute income is far easier whenever the merger joins members of the same specialty. Even then, however, doctors can slice the pie several ways. The easiest and fairest approach is simply to divide all income equally. Beyond that, the formula can get as complicated as the group desires. Some groups set aside a portion of revenues to reward doctors who top the patient satisfaction surveys. Others may reserve 10 percent of the capitation revenue and distribute it to the two or three physicians who have held down annual costs.

Most groups distribute all their revenue at the end of the year, but since the future is so uncertain, accountants advise setting some money aside to cushion unexpected blows.

Given the many issues to resolve, it's not surprising that a multipractice merger can be a laborious and often frustrating project lasting six to 12 months. In early 1994, after a year of searching for the right suitor, an orthopedic surgeon in the Hampton Roads region of northeastern Virginia had been at the negotiating table for six months and predicted another month or two would pass before closure. The surgeon, who requested anonymity because he had not yet sealed the deal, said the delays are agonizing though the result will be worth the effort.

The surgeon heads a group of eight orthopedic surgeons who work at three hospitals. They are a tight-knit group that has never made a move unless everyone agreed to it, and they split their expenses and income equally. For several decades the practice ran smoothly and income rose steadily. Then, in the 1980s, medicine changed. Medicare and Medicaid reduced fees, and major insurers soon matched the government's decreases. Within a three-year period the group's income dropped 25 percent. In 1991 capitation came to the Hampton Roads region. "We knew we had to do something, find someone to merge with," the surgeon said. "We were groping for a plan. But physicians really don't know how to do this kind of thing."

After discussions with a number of potential partners fizzled, the group found a good prospect. A practice with six orthopedic surgeons had merged in 1993 with a group of five others. Although they were all in the same specialty, the surgeons were not competitors because they served different ends of Hampton Roads. "I realized that if our group of eight hooked up with their group of 11, we'd become a force that had to be reckoned with," the surgeon said. "When this deal goes through, the 19 of us will offer more than any other orthopedic group in a region where 1.4 million people live. We'll cover all the local hospitals and offer every type of orthopedic service. Not only can we do every type of bone surgery—back, hand, pediatric—but we will also be in a position to provide subspecialty services like clinics for sports medicine, physical therapy, and total joint replacements. In addition we'll be able to afford a high-quality consultant who could show us how to market all this to HMOs or directly to businesses."

The proposed 19-surgeon group seemed likely to become a powerful force in a sizable market—if the two groups could complete the deal. A few pesky issues remained, including how many members from each group would sit on the board and how the new organization would distribute both patients and money. If the merger made so much sense, why were the negotiations taking so long? "You're dealing with strong personalities," the surgeon said. "Some of these guys are suspicious about every detail. For a long time we discussed everything as a group, but that proved unworkable." So each group chose a physician with moderate views to represent it. When this committee works out a compromise, the members take it back to their respective groups for a vote.

Despite the squabbling, the surgeon predicts the deal will go through because the physicians realize their choices are dwindling. "Small surgical groups in California are going out of business every day. It's just a matter of time until that happens here," he said. "The basic reason we're all willing to go through this protracted merger process is that we fear if we stay small, we'll be excluded. If you can't offer a wide scope of services to managed-care plans, that's what happens."

You don't have to belong to a group to enjoy the benefits of merging. The most common type of merger occurs when an individual physician decides to abandon solo practice and join a group. Since this type of arrangement is far less complicated than a multipractice merger, a physician can usually work out a deal more quickly.

For Dr. Barbara J. MacFarlane, a 41-year-old family-practice physician, merging into a group meant the difference between floundering and flourishing. In 1988 MacFarlane and her husband moved from Canada, land of a highly praised single-payer health care system, to Santa Cruz, California, about 75 miles south of San Francisco. "In Canada the government of the province you live in pays for all medical care," said MacFarlane. "When I moved here, I knew nothing about how American medicine functioned. I knew nothing about interacting with insurance companies. Absolutely nothing."

MacFarlane was not eager to plunge into the bureaucratic nightmare of medicine, American-style. She spent 15 months working for an hourly wage at an urgent-care walk-in facility. Then, in February 1990, she opened her own practice; she started with no patients and refused to accept insurance. "If you wanted to see me," MacFarlane said, "you had to pay me." As a primary-care physician with two years of orthopedic training and a master's degree in exercise physiology, she had skills that were well-suited to the community's young, active population. Individuals with sports injuries visited her office, and a back-pain rehabilitation program drew additional patients.

In 1991 MacFarlane realized her practice would remain relatively small or even shrink unless she began to deal with insurance companies. She was smart enough to see that managed care, which had already captured huge market shares elsewhere in California, would quickly extend its tentacles into Santa Cruz. She signed up with a few PPOs and studied how capitation works. In mid-1992 she contracted with five HMOs.

By that time MacFarlane's practice had grown so much that she had outgrown her rented office space and computer equipment. And she knew her problems would worsen. Her practice included 100 capitated HMO patients, a figure that she expected to soar six months later; HMOs traditionally acquire the most new members in late October, and doctors start seeing those new prepaid patients within a month or two. "I wasn't in a position to handle the growth," said MacFarlane.

The solution, she said, was obvious. She had identified a primary-care group of six internists and two family practitioners as the medical leader in the community. When she heard that the group was expanding, she told them she was interested. "If they added more doctors and became an even stronger force in town, my own practice would suffer," MacFarlane said. She knew two members of the group and grew to like the others she met during the two months of negotiations. "The personalities of the people you're working with affect so many things," said MacFarlane. "It's a critical factor."

Being buddies, however, doesn't necessarily mean doctors will win the terms they want. To achieve that goal, what they ask for must be realistic and proportional to what they add to the group. MacFarlane had plenty to offer. Her practice had grown to 1,500 patients, and she anticipated continued growth from the HMOs she had contracted with. "Look at HMO statistics and you'll see that both males and females who are enrolled prefer female physicians," she said. "It's a sore point with male doctors, but if you want your practice to grow, add female physicians." (Indeed, MacFarlane's group of prepaid patients ballooned from 100 to 1,000 within a year of joining the group.)

Furthermore, as a family practitioner MacFarlane would help attract pediatric patients, which would enhance the group's appeal to managed-care plans. Finally, her surgical training enabled her to assist during surgery, which would bring more dollars into the group's coffers.

In exchange for the value she brought to the group, MacFarlane wanted two things: to be compensated fairly and to practice medicine the way she wanted. At her request, her income is based on productivity; she keeps 40 percent of her collections, and the rest pays her share of overhead expenses. More important, she retained the right to sell her practice. "We agreed that my practice might grow just because I was part of the group, but we also agreed that a lot of patients select me because of who I am," she said. If MacFarlane does sell, she can keep 75 percent of the fee.

MacFarlane also got the flexible practice style she wanted. In a sense she is set up as a mini-cost center: the money she makes goes into her own account. Out of that she pays her nurse practitioner and keeps the remainder. In addition MacFarlane won the right to hire more people—either nurses or physicians—and to pay them a salary out of her account. "If I want to work fewer hours and pay someone to pick up the slack, I can do that," she said. So in return for all that she adds to the group, MacFarlane was able to keep much of her autonomy.

Three partners run the group, but MacFarlane doesn't mind being one of the associates; in fact, she prefers it that way. "To become a full partner I'd have to buy a piece of the group's assets," she said. "Why would I want to own one-fourth of the lab equipment and exam-room furnishings? If you can't sell it, you're stuck with it. All I want to own is the right to sell my practice, and that's what I have."

In January 1993 MacFarlane merged with the group. The maneuver enabled her to move into a larger, better equipped facility without going into debt. It also allowed her to become part of a group of doctors she describes as "fair and friendly" who are sophisticated about managed care and poised for growth. And it freed her from the management details that eat up so much of a physician's time.

But the merger did not solve one problem. As a native Canadian accustomed to a relatively simple approach to health care, she's still frustrated by the U.S. system, which is, she said, "so bureaucratic it doesn't know what it's doing."

CHAPTER *five*

Selling Your Practice

It seems as if the health care industry is on steroids: everybody believes the key to survival is to bulk up. No one can predict precisely how the medical marketplace will look in five years, but you don't need the fortune-telling powers of Nostradamus to see that the buyers of health care will reward those who provide the most services for the best price. To cope with falling fees and rising competition, a growing number of physicians feel they must belong to large, efficiently managed organizations.

What physicians used to value least, capital and management expertise, have now become highly prized resources. Since medical practices typically distribute their net income at the end of a year, they often lack cash reserves to fund expansion. And since most doctors are neither trained nor interested in the business side of a practice, they know little about designing and implementing strategic management plans. So a number of middle-aged physicians, searching for both capital and managerial skills, are doing what they once found unthinkable: selling their practices.

For any doctor who is not about to retire, selling a medical practice is a radical act, but the alternatives may be even less attractive. Doctors who want to double the size of their group could try to borrow funds from commercial banks, but loan officers want to see business plans, and they typically require the individual physicians in a group to be personally responsible for paying back the loan if the practice cannot. Furthermore, the unwise lending practices of the 1980s have made many banks gun-shy about parting with their money. Medical groups that own their buildings could use them as collateral, but banks usually limit such loans to no more than 75 percent of the appraised value of the real estate. For most practitioners in small medical buildings, that is hardly enough for a major expansion.

Before applying for multimillion-dollar loans, physicians need to ask themselves this question: Am I so confident of my economic success—despite the industry's continuing tumult—that I will risk my life savings by guaranteeing a loan for my practice? Most doctors would answer that question by posing another: Do you think I'm crazy?

Physicians who are selling their practices, particularly primary-care doctors, may draw a variety of buyers, including group practices, hospitals, and physician-management companies. A retiring doctor can sell to the highest bidder, much as if he or she were selling a house. But the decision is more complicated for physicians in their prime earning years. Large group practices offer job security and the appeal of belonging to a physician-controlled organization, yet the financial terms are not often generous. Hospitals have deeper pockets, yet many physicians who have felt mistreated by hospital administrators shudder at the thought of working for their traditional adversary. Management companies might dangle the most dollars, but a corporate culture is alien to most physicians; furthermore, working for a public company whose primary allegiance is to its shareholders—not the doctors' patients—is unpalatable.

"Doctors are not often motivated primarily by the dollars," said Alice Gosfield, herself the daughter of a doctor. "They wish they could be. They would all love to be Donald Trump when they do their deals, but that's not what runs physicians' engines. They're far more into autonomy and control. So very often the right deal for physicians is not the best deal from a business perspective."

One way to think through such a difficult decision is to distinguish which aspects of the deal are negotiable and which are not. Unless you're planning to become a hospital employee, money and autonomy are negotiable. The workplace culture, however, is not; it's simply a condition a doctor accepts or rejects. Ultimately the most important issue is the buyer's own prognosis for survival in a rapidly changing marketplace. Selling your practice to a large group in order to remain in a physician-controlled environment is only a smart move if the group also has good doctors, experience with managed-care organizations, and a well-conceived plan for growth. Selling to a hospital may work out better than you think if the hospital is solvent and well run. Selling to a management company that is underfunded, secretive about its finances, or unrealistic about its projected growth is never a good idea, whatever its positive features.

If a physician is fortunate enough to find a buyer that is financially strong, managerially adept, and deferential about clinical decisions, the two parties then must agree on a price. Getting the best deal is difficult because medical practices are valued differently than homes or businesses. Although a homeowner might jack up the asking price by repainting, last-minute cosmetics won't help physicians get better prices. Customers don't know—or much care—who owns and manages a gas station, a hardware store, or a conglomerate. But patients care who their doctors are, and many stick with physicians who move crosstown. This means that doctors possess two kinds of assets: tangible commodities such as equipment and furniture and intangibles such as reputation and customer allegiance. Physicians routinely undervalue the former and overvalue the latter.

"Physicians are often not aware that their hard assets have value even though they've been fully depreciated," said Greg B. Gates, a tax law specialist and cofounder of Gates, Moore & Company, an Atlanta health care consulting company. For example, if for tax reasons an accountant fully depreciates a $10,000 computer system purchased three years ago, it will carry no value on the practice ledger. However, a physician might use the unit for two more years. When valuing a practice, Gates advised, the accountant should redepreciate such items "on a straight-line basis over five years." In other words, the $10,000 computer loses one-fifth of its value each year; after three years, it's still worth $4,000. Accountants use lower redepreciation rates to place value on longer-lasting items such as furniture and exam tables. An alternative is to redepreciate everything in the office on a straight-line basis over 12 years. "All you're trying to do," said Gates, "is show a buyer that even though your assets may be worth zero on your books, they still have value."

Real estate is the one hard asset doctors tend to overvalue, but buyers rarely want a doctor's property. So it won't boost the sale price.

Physicians also tend to overvalue their intangible assets—income potential, patient mix, practice prestige—collectively known as goodwill. "They routinely have grandiose notions of the value of their practices," said Gosfield, "because they've devoted their lives to building them up, and they want to be paid for their life's work."

Back in the glory days of medicine, before the onset of managed care and intense government regulation, goodwill was simply an easy way to get more profit. "In many ways buyers used goodwill as a slush fund" to get the physicians they wanted, said Gosfield. A buyer and a seller, usually a hospital and doctor, would agree to an inflated price, and whatever portion of the total amount couldn't be ascribed to hard assets was labeled goodwill. "That kind of goodwill doesn't fly anymore," Gosfield said.

Increased government regulation helped bring the value of intangibles down to earth. In addition to fudging on goodwill, some hospitals and labs used to pay kickbacks to doctors for referrals of patients in Medicare and Medicaid programs. In response Congress passed the Fraud and Abuse Act, which prohibits such activity and states that violators—the briber and the bribee—can face up to five years in prison and $25,000 in fines. In the 1990s, when hospitals started acquiring medical practices at a fast clip, government regulators began to suspect that practice purchase prices might mask a hospital's payment for physicians' referrals.

In March 1993 *American Medical News*, an AMA publication, ran a page-one story headlined FEDS LOOK FOR FRAUD, ABUSE IN PRACTICE SALES. The article reprinted portions of a letter to the IRS written by D. McCarty Thornton, a top official in the inspector general's office at the Department of Health and Human Services. Thornton wrote that the government would view hospitals' paying "any amount . . . in excess of the fair market value of the hard assets of a physician practice" as actually paying for referrals in defiance of the Fraud and Abuse Act. In response hospitals began to tell physicians: "Sorry. We'd love to offer you more for your practice, but the government won't let us pay for goodwill, so you'll just have to accept a lower price."

Physicians may not be aware of it, but in February 1994, Thornton amended his remarks. In a paper prepared for the Pennsylvania Bar Institute, Thornton wrote, "There has been somewhat of an overreaction to this letter [to the IRS], because I am not saying that you can never pay for goodwill." His concern, he wrote, is "the valuation of these intangibles puffed up through creative accounting games to disguise payment for what is often one of the primary intentions of the hospital, that is, to lock in the referral stream."

How much payment for goodwill can a physician expect from a hospital? Sandra E.D. McGraw, a lawyer with the Health Care Group, a consulting firm in Plymouth Meeting, Pennsylvania, said the government's latest recommendation is that a hospital offer about the same amount as a new doctor would pay a retiring doctor for a practice.

And how much might that be? The Health Care Group publishes *The Goodwill Registry*, an annual survey of prices paid for medical practices. In 1993 payments for goodwill averaged about 30 percent of a practice's annual gross revenue. A few rules of thumb can help physicians determine whether they should expect more or less than the national average: Relationships with patients generally give primary-care practitioners a higher goodwill value than they give specialists. Doctors in urban settings garner more goodwill than those in rural areas. The higher a doctor's income compared with what competitors earn, the higher the goodwill. And the more competitors, the better; physicians who are the only members of their specialty in town will lose patients as soon as a competent competitor arrives.

An AMA publication, *Buying and Selling Medical Practices: A Valuation Guide*, lists a dozen factors that consultants evaluate to determine an appropriate goodwill figure, including the practice's financial condition, efficiency, and growth potential and the seller's reputation. Among the most important considerations, experts say, are a practice's location, the demographics of the patients, and their loyalty to the physician. In other words, if you are a primary-care physician running a well-managed practice in an affluent community brimming with young families, the value of your practice is at the top of the charts.

Although everyone wants the best price when they sell, doctors aren't placing their practices on the auction block just to rake in dollars. They don't want to get shut out of a system that is rapidly consolidating. "I understand the desire to remain on your own, but given the way the market is going, it makes more sense to align yourself with a major player," said Dr. Mark E. McCaulley, a 41-year-old internist in Steamboat Springs, Colorado.

The skiing conditions are ideal in this resort town, and McCaulley hits the slopes whenever possible, but practicing medicine in rural areas is rigorous in the best of times, and the hardships are growing. Until he sold his practice in 1993 to a group of 45 doctors in Denver, his feelings about the future were similar to those of a novice skier perched atop a steep Rocky Mountain slope. McCaulley, who had only treated fee-for-service patients, was watching the town's largest employers, the ski businesses, cut medical costs by signing up with managed-care plans. His overhead expenses were out of control, he was on call every night and weekend, and he was having a hard time recruiting a doctor to help him out.

McCaulley's troubles began in 1988, when he decided to abandon six years of solo practice and hire another internist. At the time his overhead took 55 percent of his gross revenues, so McCaulley paid his associate 45 percent of hers. One anticipated benefit of taking on a partner was the economies of scale that occur when businesses grow. He hoped the plan would reduce his overhead and enable him to pocket more of his collections. But within two years his overhead rose to 65 percent, and he was stuck with a partner who took 45 percent of her revenues.

When that associate left in 1991, McCaulley hired a replacement for $70,000 plus benefits, which added another $20,000 to the employee's cost. Managed care places such a premium on general practitioners, said McCaulley, that "internists won't look at you for less than $90,000—and that's not even very attractive to them, considering they can make $110,000 or more right out of residency." The cost of recruitment wasn't the only expense heading in the wrong direction; the salaries for his four nurses, the office manager, the receptionist, and the file clerk were climbing, and so was the rent. Meanwhile his Medicare reimbursements were dropping.

By 1991 McCaulley's income had plummeted 40 percent. "I don't have the expertise to run a business that grosses a million dollars a year, and it's silly for me to behave as though I do," he said. "I either have to pay people to do it or risk making serious mistakes." His choice was simple: watch his income continue to fall or sell the practice.

He was set to sell to a hospital in Denver when a local hospital made a better offer. But just after he broke off negotiations with the Denver buyer, the local hospital withdrew its offer. With no medical groups

Powerful Innovators

Next to excellence is the appreciation of it.

William Makepeace Thackeray

Miles is pleased to sponsor this series on Powerful Innovators to remember, recognize, and appreciate the truly remarkable achievements of the best of the medical profession.

We salute these individuals; we applaud their efforts; we remember their deeds.

More importantly, we salute and applaud the efforts today's physicians make every day.

H. Brian Allen, MD, FFPM
Director, Scientific Relations
Miles Inc.
Pharmaceutical Division

to join in his tiny community of 6,000 residents, McCaulley had few remaining options. Fortunately, Focus Health Service, a primary-care group with 10 sites in Denver, was embarking on a three-year campaign to grow from 45 to 200 doctors and cover the Denver metropolitan area as well as rural communities throughout the state. "If we want to be a player when health care reform comes down the pike, our group has to be well dispersed," said Deborah Welle-Powell, the group's administrator. "Our goal is to get to the point where the health plans can't do business without us. We don't plan on stopping when we hit 200. If we get big enough, we can approach large employers directly and bypass the insurers."

McCaulley sold his practice to Focus in December 1993, and both appear likely to benefit from the deal. McCaulley is now part of a multimillion-dollar organization eagerly pursuing managed-care contracts and implementing sound business principles. A centralized business department handles billing, collecting, contracting, and purchasing and makes management advice available. Thanks to bimonthly visits from a Focus representative, his billing systems, patient records, and staff are "in a lean, mean mode," he said, and he has hired a new associate paid by Focus. "I'm done subsidizing other doctors," said McCaulley. Moreover, he believes that belonging to the Focus group enabled him to recruit his new partner. "The salary is better than I could have offered," he said, "and the practice is more stable."

McCaulley receives a minimum guaranteed salary, and in a year he will become a shareholder with voting rights. The deal includes a "restrictive covenant," a common feature of practice sales. If he leaves the group, he is barred for three years from opening a new practice within five miles of his current office. If Focus severs its relationship with him for economic reasons, the restriction doesn't apply.

McCaulley has lost some autonomy, but he doesn't seem to mind. Focus decides, for instance, whether he needs registered nurses, medical assistants, or an on-site business manager. "That's control I was ready to give up," he said. "I'm happy to be rid of some of these pressures."

Focus will gain from the deal as well: a foothold for regional expansion and an internist who works hard to provide quality medical care to the residents of a small, remote community.

You don't have to be a solo practitioner to feel threatened by the revolutionary changes sweeping through the health care industry. The times are so uncertain that nearly every group, regardless of its size, views itself as lilliputian. No matter how big you are, conventional wisdom suggests you're not big enough.

Dr. Robert N. Schulenberg, a 51-year-old pediatrician, heads a multispecialty group of 28 physicians in Red Wing, Minnesota, 45 miles south of Minneapolis. The well-balanced practice includes pediatrics, obstetrics, gynecology, internal medicine, ophthalmology, family practice, orthopedics, urology, and general surgery. It operates from four sites within a 25-mile radius, serving Red Wing's population of 15,000 and another 45,000 in surrounding towns, accumulating revenues of $14 million a year.

In most states a powerful group like Schulenberg's would face little challenge. But in medical matters Minnesota is unusual. Large group practices dominate the medical landscape. Managed care is as strong in Minneapolis-St. Paul as it is anywhere else in the country. State legislators are working to provide health insurance to each resident. Physician groups, hospitals, and insurers are joining to form integrated delivery systems designed to handle every aspect of patient care. Only a few other places are experiencing such frenzied consolidation in the health care industry.

By car Red Wing is 45 minutes south of Minneapolis and 30 minutes north of Rochester, home of the expanding Mayo Clinic. Head east for a few miles and you cross the border into Wisconsin, where the 400-physician Marshfield Clinic has 24 satellite offices. Closer to Red Wing, a hospital corporation has gobbled up 14 primary-care clinics. "Five years ago the competition heated up, and the players were bigger than us and had a lot more assets," said Schulenberg. "One of them made a billion dollars a year in revenues." Fighting seemed foolhardy; who in his right mind would invest his life savings to take on such awesome opponents? Recruiting new doctors was not an option. The harsh weather, state taxes on medical revenue, and semirural location in a state dominated by managed care all made recruitment virtually impossible.

The group concocted a strategy that transformed its vulnerability into an asset. "We realized we were suddenly valuable," Schulenberg said. "Here we were in the center of this [medical] hotbed. We decided to get out while we still had some value. If a large organization decided to compete with us, it could take a loss for a lot longer than we could. And then we'd have no value left." Under the circumstances, deciding to sell the practice seemed more like an act of salvation than sacrifice. "None of us wanted to be investors in health care or to own medical buildings anymore," said Schulenberg.

In Minneapolis Clifford P. Fearing, the chief financial officer of the University of Minnesota Hospital and Clinic, was designing an expansion plan to fortify the teaching hospital's share of the market. Despite a force of 500 physicians and twice as many medical residents, despite money streaming in from 600,000 patient visits and 17,000 hospital admissions each year, the system's officials felt almost as insecure as Schulenberg. "Unless we get bigger—through acquisitions or by developing our own primary-care practices or by affiliating with other organizations—we will be outside the patient flow and the financial flow, and we won't be here in four or five years," said Fearing.

The system's patients come from three sources: 45 percent live in the Minneapolis-St. Paul area, 25 percent in other states, and 30 percent in outlying communities within the state, a segment of the market Fearing couldn't afford to lose. "To secure the greater Minnesota market, where Red Wing is a hub," Fearing said, "it was imperative to acquire Dr. Schulenberg's group. That way Mayo couldn't acquire it and divert all those patients and dollars to its system."

In 1992, after two years of negotiating, the two organizations completed the deal. The chief issue was not money, but who would control the group. Giving up too much control over the practice, said Schulenberg, was "a deal buster." After much wrangling they found an acceptable formula. The Red Wing group formed a new corporation, whose sole shareholder is the university hospital system. The corporation is run by a board composed of three officials from the university and three physicians from Schulenberg's group. Fearing and his colleagues have the power to veto the practice's annual budget, unbudgeted expenses in excess of $50,000, and all contracts with health plans or businesses. The practice has its own physician executive committee that oversees daily operations.

The Red Wing practice relinquished some autonomy, but the gains outweigh the losses. By tapping in to the university's teaching program, the group solved its recruiting problems and has grown to 38 doctors. Thanks to capital provided by the university, the practice will move into a new hospital and clinic on a 300-acre site. The group sold its four buildings to the university, assets the physicians were happy to unload since they hadn't appreciated much. "We would have been better off if we'd bought shares of Microsoft," said Schulenberg. And since the group owns no assets, it no longer requires a $30,000 buy-in fee from new physicians, which had also hampered recruitment.

Now that the practice is set up as a not-for-profit organization, which protects the university's tax-exempt status, the group is stockpiling capital for continued expansion. "We were going in that direction anyway," said Schulenberg. "The clinics that will survive are those that accumulate assets; they can respond to changes in the marketplace without borrowing money." With that capital the group can grow by acquiring small practices of three to five doctors.

Schulenberg knows he probably could have received more money from other buyers; when he was negotiating with the university, he was approached by a member of a hospital corporation who said, "Anything they'll do, we'll do even better." But Schulenberg's advice is to focus on the partner, not the price. Hospital corporations "dangle some fairly enchanting numbers in front of you," he said, "but you better make sure you want to work for them." Furthermore, he added, the marketplace is changing so quickly that some outfits that appear strong today may go out of business within a few years. "The University of Minnesota," he concluded, "will be here forever."

Medical groups and hospitals aren't the only ones busily buying doctors' practices. A handful of publicly held companies do nothing but invest in and manage physician practices. Their targets are usually groups of 10 or more doctors in demographically attractive locations. These physician-management companies typically buy such practice assets as equipment, accounts receivable, and, occasionally, real estate. They pump capital into an acquired practice so it can expand, supply management expertise so it runs more efficiently, negotiate contracts with vendors and insurers to lower overhead, and collect a management fee, usually about 7 percent of the practice's revenue.

The oldest and largest of these companies is PhyCor, based in Nashville, which owns 19 practices in 12 states. Joseph C. Hutts, the president and chief executive officer, said PhyCor is shopping for multispecialty practices with at least 25 physicians, though it will acquire groups of two to five primary-care physicians "who might be interested in joining a clinic we already have." Why would physicians want to sell to a public company, which presumably has to please its shareholders first? Here's Hutts's sales pitch: "If you're in a physician-driven organization that can attain the critical mass in a marketplace to dominate a network, then you're in a strong position with the insurers, and you can negotiate a much stronger deal."

To Dr. James Saalfield, a 49-year-old urologist who heads a 43-doctor multispecialty group in Texas, Hutts's strength-in-numbers argument made sense. Before selling to PhyCor in 1993, the Medical-Surgical Clinic of Irving was experiencing problems that many practices face. About 60 percent of the group's patients were covered by traditional fee-for-service insurers, and the rest were covered by Medicare or discounted PPO plans. The clinic had no capitated contracts, a situation it knew would soon change. Its percentage of indemnity patients, though still relatively high, was dropping fast.

To make up for decreasing revenue, the group tried offering as many services as possible, operating a pathology lab, a radiology deparment, and an urgent-care clinic seven days a week. Unfortunately, instead of enhancing the bottom line, the services were draining funds. "We were like the federal government," said Saalfield. "We were spending more than we were taking in." In addition, some of the group's highest producing doctors quit when they couldn't agree about compensation, and recruiting efforts weren't working. "We were floundering," Saalfield said.

The clinic was just what PhyCor was looking for. It was the only large multispecialty practice in the Dallas-Forth Worth megalopolis, and the group's practitioners earned more than their competitors. In 1992 some PhyCor officials visited the clinic and recommended what the group should do to become more competitive: hire an occupational physician, offer physical therapy, buy a CT scanner, and upgrade the urgent-care facility. Join us, PhyCor's officials said, and we'll help you make those improvements. The group's response to PhyCor's offer of cash and stock—its standard way of financing acquisitions—was a flat no. "We didn't want any stock," said Saalfield, "because if PhyCor went belly-up, the stock would be worthless." Furthermore, the physicians were not yet ready for such a change. They thanked the visitors for their advice and broke off negotiations, figuring they could implement the plans themselves. Before long, Saalfield said, the group realized that "we weren't going to accomplish any of these things because we were all too busy practicing medicine—and we didn't have the resources or the expertise."

A year later they called PhyCor to reopen the talks, still opting for an all-cash offer. PhyCor agreed. A large lump-sum payment, the amount of which neither side will divulge, was divided equally among the physicians. A policy board composed of three PhyCor officials and three of the clinic's doctors runs the operation. Bulk purchasing contracts from PhyCor's central business office have already saved the group $150,000 in lab costs and many thousands more in malpractice policies that cost less yet provide greater coverage. PhyCor bought the group a CT scanner for $800,000, and as with all new services that PhyCor funds, the profits are split 50-50. The other services that PhyCor had suggested are also now in place.

Because it lays out so much capital, PhyCor demands long-term commitments from physicians. The agreement between the company and the clinic runs for 30 years. During the life of the contract, if a doctor leaves the clinic and opens a practice within 10 miles of the group's current location, his or her share of the up-front payment must be returned to PhyCor. "It's a golden handcuff," said Saalfield.

The clinic's physicians don't seem to mind. "It's a business. We can still practice medicine the way we want to. Phycor offers a good vision of the future, it's honest, and it's done everything it promised," said Saalfield. "The only downside is that you have to keep growing and adding new services to keep generating money, but these days you have to do that anyway."

conclusion

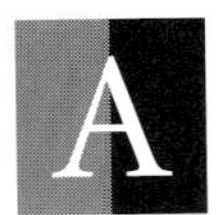

A natural response to the upheaval buffeting the health care industry is to proceed cautiously. The temptation is to hunker down and wait for the confusion to subside.

Unfortunately the luxury of playing for time no longer exists. When HMOs arrive in a community or when fee-for-service insurers switch to capitation, physicians who stay on the sidelines do so at their own peril. First they run the risk of being told that an HMO's panel of providers is closed to new members. At that point doctors have lost access to the patients who have enrolled in the plans. In addition, stalling keeps doctors one step behind competitors who are becoming acquainted with the nuances of managed-care contracting as well as the economics of capitation.

Similarly, if physicians in solo practice or in small groups postpone affiliating with a larger group until the dust settles, they're likely to find themselves out of the loop altogether. Robert C. Bohlmann, head of consulting at the Medical Group Management Association, predicts "a substantial shakeout in the marketplace within three years." Negotiating a merger often requires six to 12 months, and hammering out the details of a sale can take even longer. Add to that the time it takes to find the right partner, and you can see that while there's no need to act hastily, it is imperative to act.

Physicians who are willing to experiment with managed care now, who understand the processes of networks and mergers, of negotiations and sales, will have the surest footing later on. They will know how to strengthen their position in the marketplace, enabling them to attain a basic yet increasingly elusive goal: the opportunity to treat patients in the manner they think best.

Additional Copies

To order copies of *On Your Terms* for friends or colleagues, please write to The Grand Rounds Press, Whittle Books, 333 Main St., Knoxville, Tenn. 37902. Please include the recipient's name, mailing address, and, where applicable, primary specialty and ME number.

For a single copy, please enclose a check for $21.95 plus $3.50 for postage and handling, payable to The Grand Rounds Press. Quantities may be limited. Discounts apply to bulk orders when available. To order by phone using your MasterCard or Visa card, please call 800-765-5889.

Also available, at the same price, are copies of the previous books from The Grand Rounds Press:

The Doctor Watchers by Spencer Vibbert
The New Genetics by Leon Jaroff
Surgeon Koop by Gregg Easterbrook
Inside Medical Washington by James H. Sammons, M.D.
Medicine For Sale by Richard Currey
The Doctor Dilemma by Gerald R. Weissmann, M.D.
Taking Care of Your Own by Perri Klass, M.D.
The Logic of Health-Care Reform by Paul Starr
Raising the Dead by Richard Selzer
Malpractice Solutions by James Rosenblum
What Works by Spencer Vibbert

MD/2000:
Revolution by Russell C. Coile Jr.
Decision Point by Michael B. Guthrie, M.D.

Please allow four weeks for delivery.
Tennessee residents must add 8 1/4 percent sales tax.

PRESCRIBING INFORMATION APPENDIX

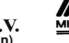

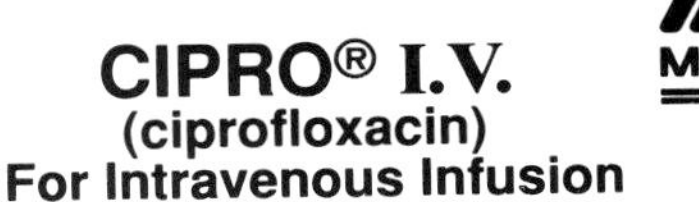

CIPRO® I.V.
(ciprofloxacin)
For Intravenous Infusion

PZ100736

DESCRIPTION

Cipro® I.V. (ciprofloxacin) is a synthetic broad-spectrum antimicrobial agent for intravenous (iv) administration. Ciprofloxacin, a fluoroquinolone, is 1-cyclopropyl-6-fluoro-1, 4-dihydro-4-oxo-7-(1-piperazinyl)-3-quinolinecarboxylic acid. Its empirical formula is $C_{17}H_{18}FN_3O_3$ and its chemical structure is:

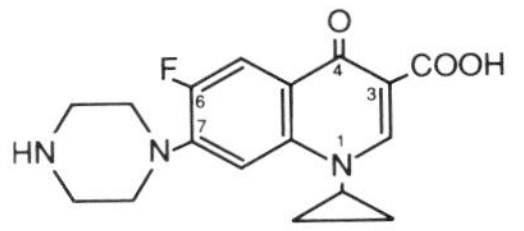

Ciprofloxacin is a faint to light yellow crystalline powder with a molecular weight of 331.4. It is soluble in dilute (0.1N) hydrochloric acid and is practically insoluble in water and ethanol. Ciprofloxacin differs from other quinolones in that it has a fluorine atom at the 6-position, a piperazine moiety at the 7-position, and a cyclopropyl ring at the 1-position. Cipro® I.V. solutions are available as 1.0% aqueous concentrates, which are intended for dilution prior to administration, and as a 0.2% ready-for-use infusion solution in 5% Dextrose Injection. All formulas contain lactic acid as a solubilizing agent and hydrochloric acid for pH adjustment. The pH range for the 1.0% aqueous concentrates in vials is 3.3 to 3.9. The pH range for the 0.2% ready-for-use infusion solutions is 3.5 to 4.6.

The plastic container is fabricated from a specially formulated polyvinyl chloride. Solutions in contact with the plastic container can leach out certain of its chemical components in very small amounts within the expiration period, e.g., di(2-ethylhexyl) phthalate (DEHP), up to 5 parts per million. The suitability of the plastic has been confirmed in tests in animals according to USP biological tests for plastic containers as well as by tissue culture toxicity studies.

CLINICAL PHARMACOLOGY

Following 60-minute intravenous infusions of 200 mg and 400 mg ciprofloxacin to normal volunteers, the mean maximum serum concentrations achieved were 2.1 and 4.6 µg/mL, respectively; the concentrations at 12 hours were 0.1 and 0.2 µg/mL, respectively.

Steady-state Ciprofloxacin Serum Concentrations (µg/mL) After 60-minute IV Infusions q 12 h.

	Time after starting the infusion					
Dose	**30 min.**	**1 hr**	**3 hr**	**6 hr**	**8 hr**	**12 hr**
200 mg	1.7	2.1	0.6	0.3	0.2	0.1
400 mg	3.7	4.6	1.3	0.7	0.5	0.2

The pharmacokinetics of ciprofloxacin are linear over the dose range of 200 to 400 mg administered intravenously. The serum elimination half-life is approximately 5–6 hours and the total clearance is around 35 L/hr. Comparison of the pharmacokinetic parameters following the 1st and 5th iv dose on a q 12 h regimen indicates no evidence of drug accumulation.

The absolute bioavailability of oral ciprofloxacin is within a range of 70–80% with no substantial loss by first pass metabolism. An intravenous infusion of 400 mg ciprofloxacin given over 60 minutes every 12 hours has been shown to produce an area under the serum concentration time curve (AUC) equivalent to that produced by a 500 mg oral dose given every 12 hours. A 400 mg iv dose administered over 60 minutes every 12 hours results in a C_{max} similar to that observed with a 750 mg oral dose. An infusion of 200 mg ciprofloxacin given every 12 hours produces an AUC equivalent to that produced by a 250 mg oral dose given every 12 hours.

After intravenous administration, approximately 50% to 70% of the dose is excreted in the urine as unchanged drug. Following a 200 mg iv dose, concentrations in the urine usually exceed 200 µg/mL 0–2 hours after dosing and are generally greater than 15 µg/mL 8–12 hours after dosing. Following a 400 mg iv dose, urine concentrations generally exceed 400 µg/mL 0–2 hours after dosing and are usually greater than 30 µg/mL 8–12 hours after dosing. The renal clearance is approximately 22 L/hr. The urinary excretion of ciprofloxacin is virtually complete by 24 hours after dosing.

Co-administration of probenecid with ciprofloxacin results in about a 50% reduction in the ciprofloxacin renal clearance and a 50% increase in its concentration in the systemic circulation. Although bile concentrations of ciprofloxacin are severalfold higher than serum concentrations after intravenous dosing, only a small amount of the administered dose (<1%) is recovered from the bile as unchanged drug. Approximately 15% of an iv dose is recovered from the feces within 5 days after dosing.

After iv administration, three metabolites of ciprofloxacin have been identified in human urine which together account for approximately 10% of the intravenous dose.

In patients with reduced renal function, the half-life of ciprofloxacin is slightly prolonged and dosage adjustments may be required. (See DOSAGE AND ADMINISTRATION.)

In preliminary studies in patients with stable chronic liver cirrhosis, no significant changes in ciprofloxacin pharmacokinetics have been observed. However, the kinetics of ciprofloxacin in patients with acute hepatic insufficiency have not been fully elucidated.

The binding of ciprofloxacin to serum proteins is 20 to 40%.

After intravenous administration, ciprofloxacin is present in saliva, nasal and bronchial secretions, sputum, skin blister fluid, lymph, peritoneal fluid, bile and prostatic secretions. It has also been detected in the lung, skin, fat, muscle, cartilage and bone. Although the drug diffuses into cerebrospinal fluid (CSF), CSF concentrations are generally less than 10% of peak serum concentrations. Levels of the drug in the aqueous and vitreous chambers of the eye are lower than in serum.

Microbiology: Ciprofloxacin has *in vitro* activity against a wide range of gram-negative and gram-positive organisms. The bactericidal action of ciprofloxacin results from interference with the enzyme DNA gyrase which is needed for the synthesis of bacterial DNA.

Ciprofloxacin has been shown to be active against most strains of the following organisms both *in vitro* and in clinical infections. (See INDICATIONS AND USAGE section.)

Gram-positive bacteria
Enterococcus faecalis (Many strains are only moderately susceptible)
Staphylococcus aureus
Staphylococcus epidermidis
Streptococcus pneumoniae
Streptococcus pyogenes

Gram-negative bacteria
Citrobacter diversus
Citrobacter freundii
Enterobacter cloacae
Escherichia coli
Haemophilus influenzae
Haemophilus parainfluenzae
Klebsiella pneumoniae
Morganella morganii
Proteus mirabilis
Proteus vulgaris
Providencia rettgeri
Providencia stuartii
Pseudomonas aeruginosa
Serratia marcescens

Ciprofloxacin has been shown to be active *in vitro* against most strains of the following organisms; however, *the clinical significance of these data is unknown.*

Gram-positive bacteria
Staphylococcus haemolyticus
Staphylococcus hominis
Staphylococcus saprophyticus

Gram-negative bacteria
Acinetobacter calcoaceticus
Aeromonas caviae
Aeromonas hydrophila
Brucella melitensis
Campylobacter coli
Campylobacter jejuni
Edwardsiella tarda
Enterobacter aerogenes
Haemophilus ducreyi
Klebsiella oxytoca
Legionella pneumophila
Moraxella (Branhamella) catarrhalis
Neisseria gonorrhoeae
Neisseria meningitidis
Pasteurella multocida
Salmonella enteritidis
Salmonella typhi
Shigella flexneri
Shigella sonnei
Vibrio cholerae
Vibrio parahaemolyticus
Vibrio vulnificus
Yersinia enterocolitica

Other organisms
Chlamydia trachomatis (only moderately susceptible)
Mycobacterium tuberculosis (only moderately susceptible)

Most strains of *Pseudomonas cepacia* and some strains of *Pseudomonas maltophilia* are resistant to ciprofloxacin as are most anaerobic bacteria, including *Bacteroides fragilis* and *Clostridium difficile.*

Ciprofloxacin is slightly less active when tested at acidic pH. The inoculum size has little effect when tested *in vitro.* The minimum bactericidal concentration (MBC) generally does not exceed the minimum inhibitory concentration (MIC) by more than a factor of 2. Resistance to ciprofloxacin *in vitro* usually develops slowly (multiple-step mutation).

Ciprofloxacin does not cross-react with other antimicrobial agents such as beta-lactams or aminoglycosides; therefore, organisms resistant to these drugs may be susceptible to ciprofloxacin.

In vitro studies have shown that additive activity often results when ciprofloxacin is combined with other antimicrobial agents such as beta-lactams, aminoglycosides, clindamycin, or metronidazole. Synergy has been reported particularly with the combination of ciprofloxacin and a beta-lactam; antagonism is observed only rarely.

Susceptibility Tests

Diffusion Techniques: Quantitative methods that require measurement of zone diameters give the most precise estimates of antibiotic susceptibility. One such procedure recommended for use with the 5-µg ciprofloxacin disk is the National Committee for Clinical Laboratory Standards (NCCLS) approved procedure (M2-A4--Performance Standards for Antimicrobial Disc Susceptibility Tests 1990). Only a 5-µg ciprofloxacin disk should be used, and it should not be used for testing susceptibility to less active quinolones; there are no suitable surrogate disks.

Results of laboratory tests using 5-µg ciprofloxacin disks should be interpreted using the following criteria:

Zone Diameter (mm)	Interpretation
≥ 21	(S) Susceptible
16 - 20	(MS) Moderately Susceptible
≤ 15	(R) Resistant

Dilution Techniques: Broth and agar dilution methods, such as those recommended by the NCCLS (M7-A2--Methods for Dilution Antimicrobial Susceptibility Tests for Bacteria that Grow Aerobically 1990), may be used to determine the minimum inhibitory concentration (MIC) of ciprofloxacin. MIC test results should be interpreted according to the following criteria:

MIC (µg/mL)	Interpretation
≤ 1	(S) Susceptible
2	(MS) Moderately Susceptible
≥ 4	(R) Resistant

For any susceptibility test, a report of "susceptible" indicates that the pathogen is likely to be inhibited by generally achievable blood levels. A report of "resistant" indicates that the pathogen is not likely to respond. A report of "moderately susceptible" indicates that the pathogen is expected to be susceptible to ciprofloxacin if high doses are used, or if the infection is confined to tissues and fluids in which high ciprofloxacin levels are attained.

The Quality Control (QC) strains should have the following assigned daily ranges for ciprofloxacin.

QC Strains	Disk Zone Diameter (mm)	MIC (µg/mL)
S. aureus (ATCC 25923)	22 – 30	——
S. aureus (ATCC 29213)	——	0.12 – 0.5
E. coli (ATCC 25922)	30 – 40	0.004 – 0.015
P. aeruginosa (ATCC 27853)	25 – 33	0.25 – 1.0
E. faecalis (ATCC 29212)	——	0.25 – 2.0

INDICATIONS AND USAGE

Cipro® I.V. is indicated for the treatment of infections caused by susceptible strains of the designated microorganisms in the conditions listed below when the intravenous administration offers a route of administration advantageous to the patient:

Urinary Tract Infections – mild, moderate, severe and complicated infections caused by *Escherichia coli*, (including cases with secondary bacteremia), *Klebsiella pneumoniae* subspecies *pneumoniae, Enterobacter cloacae, Serratia marcescens, Proteus mirabilis, Providencia rettgeri, Morganella morganii, Citrobacter diversus, Citrobacter freundii, Pseudomonas aeruginosa, Staphylococcus epidermidis*, and *Enterococcus faecalis*.

Cipro® I.V. is also indicated for the treatment of mild to moderate lower respiratory tract infections, skin and skin structure infections and bone and joint infections due to the organisms listed in each section below. In severe and complicated lower respiratory tract infections, skin and skin structure infections and bone and joint infections, safety and effectiveness of the iv formulation have not been established.

Lower Respiratory Infections – mild to moderate infections caused by *Escherichia coli, Klebsiella pneumoniae* subspecies *pneumoniae, Enterobacter cloacae, Proteus mirabilis, Pseudomonas aeruginosa, Haemophilus influenzae, Haemophilus parainfluenzae*, and *Streptococcus pneumoniae*.

Skin and Skin Structure Infections – mild to moderate infections caused by *Escherichia coli, Klebsiella pneumoniae* subspecies *pneumoniae, Enterobacter cloacae, Proteus mirabilis, Proteus vulgaris, Providencia stuartii, Morganella morganii, Citrobacter freundii, Pseudomonas aeruginosa, Staphylococcus aureus, Staphylococcus epidermidis*, and *Streptococcus pyogenes*.

Bone and Joint Infections – mild to moderate infections caused by *Enterobacter cloacae, Serratia marcescens*, and *Pseudomonas aeruginosa*.

If anaerobic organisms are suspected of contributing to the infection, appropriate therapy should be administered.

Appropriate culture and susceptibility tests should be performed before treatment in order to isolate and identify organisms causing infection and to determine their susceptibility to ciprofloxacin. Therapy with Cipro® I.V. may be initiated before results of these tests are known; once results become available, appropriate therapy should be continued.

As with other drugs, some strains of *Pseudomonas aeruginosa* may develop resistance fairly rapidly during treatment with ciprofloxacin. Culture and susceptibility testing performed periodically during therapy will provide information not only on the therapeutic effect of the antimicrobial agent but also on the possible emergence of bacterial resistance.

CONTRAINDICATIONS

Cipro® I.V. (ciprofloxacin) is contraindicated in persons with a history of hypersensitivity to ciprofloxacin or any member of the quinolone class of antimicrobial agents.

WARNINGS

THE SAFETY AND EFFECTIVENESS OF CIPROFLOXACIN IN CHILDREN, ADOLESCENTS (LESS THAN 18 YEARS OF AGE), PREGNANT WOMEN, AND LACTATING WOMEN HAVE NOT BEEN ESTABLISHED. (SEE PRECAUTIONS - PEDIATRIC USE, PREGNANCY AND NURSING MOTHERS SUBSECTIONS.) Ciprofloxacin causes lameness in immature dogs. Histopathological examination of the weight-bearing joints of these dogs revealed permanent lesions of the cartilage. Related quinolone-class drugs also produce erosions of cartilage of weight-bearing joints and other signs of arthropathy in immature animals of various species. (See ANIMAL PHARMACOLOGY.)

Convulsions have been reported in patients receiving ciprofloxacin. Convulsions, increased intracranial pressure, and toxic psychosis have been reported in patients receiving ciprofloxacin and other drugs of this class. Quinolones may also cause central nervous system (CNS) stimulation which may lead to tremors, restlessness, lightheadedness, confusion and hallucinations. If these reactions occur in patients receiving ciprofloxacin, the drug should be discontinued and appropriate measures instituted. As with all quinolones, ciprofloxacin should be used with caution in patients with known or suspected CNS disorders, such as severe cerebral arteriosclerosis, epilepsy, and other factors that predispose to seizures. (See ADVERSE REACTIONS.)

SERIOUS AND FATAL REACTIONS HAVE BEEN REPORTED IN PATIENTS RECEIVING CONCURRENT ADMINISTRATION OF INTRAVENOUS CIPROFLOXACIN AND THEOPHYLLINE. These reactions have included cardiac arrest, seizure, status epilepticus and respiratory failure. Although similar serious adverse events have been reported in patients receiving theophylline alone, the possibility that these reactions may be potentiated by ciprofloxacin cannot be eliminated. If concomitant use cannot be avoided, serum levels of theophylline should be monitored and dosage adjustments made as appropriate.

Serious and occasionally fatal hypersensitivity (anaphylactic) reactions, some following the first dose, have been reported in patients receiving quinolone therapy. Some reactions were accompanied by cardiovascular collapse, loss of consciousness, tingling, pharyngeal or facial edema, dyspnea, urticaria, and itching. Only a few patients had a history of hypersensitivity reactions. Serious anaphylactic reactions require immediate emergency treatment with epinephrine and other resuscitation measures, including oxygen, intravenous fluids, intravenous antihistamines, corticosteroids, pressor amines and airway management, as clinically indicated.

Severe hypersensitivity reactions characterized by rash, fever, eosinophilia, jaundice, and hepatic necrosis with fatal outcome have also been reported extremely rarely in patients receiving ciprofloxacin along with other drugs. The possibility that these reactions were related to ciprofloxacin cannot be excluded. Ciprofloxacin should be discontinued at the first appearance of a skin rash or any other sign of hypersensitivity.

Pseudomembranous colitis has been reported with nearly all antibacterial agents, including ciprofloxacin, and may range in severity from mild to life-threatening. Therefore, it is important to consider this diagnosis in patients who present with diarrhea subsequent to the administration of antibacterial agents.

Treatment with antibacterial agents alters the normal flora of the colon and may permit overgrowth of clostridia. Studies indicate that a toxin produced by *Clostridium difficile* is one primary cause of "antibiotic-associated colitis".

After the diagnosis of pseudomembranous colitis has been established, therapeutic measures should be initiated. Mild cases of pseudomembranous colitis usually respond to drug discontinuation alone. In moderate to severe cases, consideration should be given to management with fluids and electrolytes, protein supplementation and treatment with an antibacterial drug effective against *C. difficile*.

PRECAUTIONS

General: INTRAVENOUS CIPROFLOXACIN SHOULD BE ADMINISTERED BY SLOW INFUSION OVER A PERIOD OF 60 MINUTES. Local iv site reactions have been reported with the intravenous administration of ciprofloxacin. These reactions are more frequent if infusion time is 30 minutes or less or if small veins of the hand are used. (See ADVERSE REACTIONS.)

Crystals of ciprofloxacin have been observed rarely in the urine of human subjects but more frequently in the urine of laboratory animals, which is usually alkaline. (See ANIMAL PHARMACOLOGY.) Crystalluria related to ciprofloxacin has been reported only rarely in humans because human urine is usually acidic. Alkalinity of the urine should be avoided in patients receiving ciprofloxacin. Patients should be well hydrated to prevent the formation of highly concentrated urine.

Alteration of the dosage regimen is necessary for patients with impairment of renal function. (See DOSAGE AND ADMINISTRATION.)

Moderate to severe phototoxicity manifested by an exaggerated sunburn reaction has been observed in some patients who were exposed to direct sunlight while receiving some members of the quinolone class of drugs. Excessive sunlight should be avoided.

As with any potent drug, periodic assessment of organ system functions, including renal, hepatic, and hematopoietic, is advisable during prolonged therapy.

Information for Patients: Patients should be advised that ciprofloxacin may be associated with hypersensitivity reactions, even following a single dose, and to discontinue the drug at the first sign of a skin rash or other allergic reaction.

Ciprofloxacin may cause dizziness and lightheadedness; therefore, patients should know how they react to this drug before they operate an automobile or machinery or engage in activities requiring mental alertness or coordination.

Patients should be advised that ciprofloxacin may increase the effects of theophylline and caffeine. There is a possibility of caffeine accumulation when products containing caffeine are consumed while taking quinolones.

Drug Interactions: As with other quinolones, concurrent administration of ciprofloxacin with theophylline may lead to elevated serum concentrations of theophylline and prolongation of its elimination half-life. This may result in increased risk of theophylline-related adverse reactions. (See WARNINGS.) If concomitant use cannot be avoided, serum levels of theophylline should be monitored and dosage adjustments made as appropriate.

Some quinolones, including ciprofloxacin, have also been shown to interfere with the metabolism of caffeine. This may lead to reduced clearance of caffeine and a prolongation of its serum half-life.

Some quinolones, including ciprofloxacin, have been associated with transient elevations in serum creatinine in patients receiving cyclosporine concomitantly.

Quinolones have been reported to enhance the effects of the oral anticoagulant warfarin or its derivatives. When these products are administered concomitantly, prothrombin time or other suitable coagulation tests should be closely monitored.

Probenecid interferes with renal tubular secretion of ciprofloxacin and produces an increase in the level of ciprofloxacin in the serum. This should be considered if patients are receiving both drugs concomitantly.

As with other broad-spectrum antimicrobial agents, prolonged use of ciprofloxacin may result in overgrowth of nonsusceptible organisms. Repeated evaluation of the patient's condition and microbial susceptibility testing are essential. If superinfection occurs during therapy, appropriate measures should be taken.

Carcinogenesis, Mutagenesis, Impairment of Fertility: Eight *in vitro* mutagenicity tests have been conducted with ciprofloxacin. Test results are listed below:

- *Salmonella*/Microsome Test (Negative)
- *E. coli* DNA Repair Assay (Negative)
- Mouse Lymphoma Cell Forward Mutation Assay (Positive)
- Chinese Hamster V_{79} Cell HGPRT Test (Negative)
- Syrian Hamster Embryo Cell Transformation Assay (Negative)
- *Saccharomyces cerevisiae* Point Mutation Assay (Negative)
- *Saccharomyces cerevisiae* Mitotic Crossover and Gene Conversion Assay (Negative)
- Rat Hepatocyte DNA Repair Assay (Positive)

Thus, two of the eight tests were positive, but results of the following three *in vivo* test systems gave negative results:

- Rat Hepatocyte DNA Repair Assay
- Micronucleus Test (Mice)
- Dominant Lethal Test (Mice)

Long-term carcinogenicity studies in mice and rats have been completed. After daily oral dosing for up to 2 years, there is no evidence that ciprofloxacin has any carcinogenic or tumorigenic effects in these species.

Pregnancy: Teratogenic Effects. Pregnancy Category C: Reproduction studies have been performed in rats and mice at doses up to 6 times the usual daily human dose and have revealed no evidence of impaired fertility or harm to the fetus due to ciprofloxacin. In rabbits, ciprofloxacin (30 and 100 mg/kg orally) produced gastrointestinal disturbances resulting in maternal weight loss and an increased incidence of abortion. No teratogenicity was observed at either dose. After intravenous administration of doses up to 20 mg/kg, no maternal toxicity was produced, and no embryotoxicity or teratogenicity was observed. There are, however, no adequate and well-controlled studies in pregnant women. Ciprofloxacin should be used during pregnancy only if the potential benefit justifies the potential risk to the fetus. (See WARNINGS.)

Nursing Mothers: Ciprofloxacin is excreted in human milk. Because of the potential for serious adverse reactions in infants nursing from mothers taking ciprofloxacin, a decision should be made either to discontinue nursing or to discontinue the drug, taking into account the importance of the drug to the mother.

Pediatric Use: Safety and effectiveness in children and adolescents less than 18 years of age have not been established. Ciprofloxacin causes arthropathy in juvenile animals. (See WARNINGS.)

ADVERSE REACTIONS

The most frequently reported events, without regard to drug relationship, among patients treated with intravenous ciprofloxacin were nausea, diarrhea, central nervous system disturbance, local iv site reactions, abnormalities of liver associated enzymes (hepatic enzymes) and eosinophilia. Headache, restlessness and rash were also noted in greater than 1% of patients treated with the most common doses of ciprofloxacin.

Local iv site reactions have been reported with the intravenous administration of ciprofloxacin. These reactions are more frequent if the infusion time is 30 minutes or less. These may appear as local skin reactions which resolve rapidly upon completion of the infusion. Subsequent intravenous administration is not contraindicated unless the reactions recur or worsen.

Additional events, without regard to drug relationship or route of administration, that occurred in 1% or less of ciprofloxacin courses are listed below:

GASTROINTESTINAL: ileus; jaundice; gastrointestinal bleeding; *C. difficile* associated diarrhea; pseudomembranous colitis; pancreatitis; hepatic necrosis; intestinal perforation; dyspepsia; epigastric or abdominal pain; vomiting; constipation; oral ulceration; oral candidiasis; mouth dryness; anorexia; dysphagia; flatulence.

CENTRAL NERVOUS SYSTEM: convulsive seizures, paranoia, toxic psychosis, depression, dysphasia, phobia, depersonalization, manic reaction, unresponsiveness, ataxia, confusion, hallucinations, dizziness, lightheadedness, paresthesia, anxiety, tremor, insomnia, nightmares, weakness, drowsiness, irritability, malaise, lethargy.
SKIN/HYPERSENSITIVITY: anaphylactic reactions; erythema multiforme/-Stevens-Johnson syndrome; exfoliative dermatitis; toxic epidermal necrolysis; vasculitis; angioedema; edema of the lips, face, neck, conjunctivae, hands or lower extremities; purpura; fever; chills; flushing; pruritus; urticaria; cutaneous candidiasis; vesicles; increased perspiration; hyperpigmentation; erythema nodosum; photosensitivity.
Allergic reactions ranging from urticaria to anaphylactic reactions have been reported. (See WARNINGS.)
SPECIAL SENSES: decreased visual acuity, blurred vision, disturbed vision (flashing lights, change in color perception, overbrightness of lights, diplopia), eye pain, anosmia, hearing loss, tinnitus, nystagmus, a bad taste.
MUSCULOSKELETAL: joint pain; jaw, arm or back pain; joint stiffness; neck and chest pain; achiness; flareup of gout.
RENAL/UROGENITAL: renal failure, interstitial nephritis, hemorrhagic cystitis, renal calculi, frequent urination, acidosis, urethral bleeding, polyuria, urinary retention, gynecomastia, candiduria, vaginitis. Crystalluria, cylindruria, hematuria, and albuminuria have also been reported.
CARDIOVASCULAR: cardiovascular collapse, cardiopulmonary arrest, myocardial infarction, arrhythmia, tachycardia, palpitation, cerebral thrombosis, syncope, cardiac murmur, hypertension, hypotension, angina pectoris.
RESPIRATORY: respiratory arrest, pulmonary embolism, dyspnea, pulmonary edema, respiratory distress, pleural effusion, hemoptysis, epistaxis, hiccough.
IV INFUSION SITE: thrombophlebitis, burning, pain, pruritus, paresthesia, erythema, swelling.

Also reported were agranulocytosis, prolongation of prothrombin time and possible exacerbation of myasthenia gravis.

Many of these events were described as only mild or moderate in severity, abated soon after the drug was discontinued and required no treatment.

In several instances, nausea, vomiting, tremor, irritability or palpitation were judged by investigators to be related to elevated serum levels of theophylline possibly as a result of drug interaction with ciprofloxacin.

Adverse Laboratory Changes: The most frequently reported changes in laboratory parameters with intravenous ciprofloxacin therapy, without regard to drug relationship, were:

Hepatic	—	Elevations of AST (SGOT), ALT (SGPT), alkaline phosphatase, LDH and serum bilirubin.
Hematologic	—	Elevated eosinophil and platelet counts, decreased platelet counts, hemoglobin and/or hematocrit.
Renal	—	Elevations of serum creatinine, BUN, uric acid.
Other	—	Elevations of serum creatine phosphokinase, serum theophylline (in patients receiving theophylline concomitantly), blood glucose, and triglycerides.

Other changes occurring infrequently were: decreased leukocyte count, elevated atypical lymphocyte count, immature WBCs, elevated serum calcium, elevation of serum gamma-glutamyl transpeptidase (γ GT), decreased BUN, decreased uric acid, decreased total serum protein, decreased serum albumin, decreased serum potassium, elevated serum potassium, elevated serum cholesterol.

Other changes occurring rarely during administration of ciprofloxacin were: elevation of serum amylase, decrease of blood glucose, pancytopenia, leukocytosis, elevated sedimentation rate, change in serum phenytoin, decreased prothrombin time, hemolytic anemia, and bleeding diathesis.

OVERDOSAGE

In the event of acute overdosage, the patient should be carefully observed and given supportive treatment. Adequate hydration must be maintained. Only a small amount of ciprofloxacin (<10%) is removed from the body after hemodialysis or peritoneal dialysis.

DOSAGE AND ADMINISTRATION

The recommended adult dosage for urinary tract infections of mild to moderate severity is 200 mg every 12 hours. For severe or complicated urinary tract infections the recommended dosage is 400 mg every 12 hours.

The recommended adult dosage for lower respiratory tract infections, skin and skin structure infections and bone and joint infections of mild to moderate severity is 400 mg every 12 hours.

The determination of dosage for any particular patient must take into consideration the severity and nature of the infection, the susceptibility of the causative organism, the integrity of the patient's host-defense mechanisms and the status of renal and hepatic function.

DOSAGE GUIDELINES

Location of Infection	Type or Severity	Intravenous Unit Dose	Frequency	Daily Dose
Urinary tract	Mild/ Moderate	200 mg	q 12 h	400 mg
	Severe/ Complicated	400 mg	q 12 h	800 mg
Lower Respiratory tract; Skin and Skin Structure; Bone and Joint	Mild/ Moderate	400 mg	q 12 h	800 mg

Cipro® I.V. should be administered by intravenous infusion over a period of 60 minutes.

The duration of treatment depends upon the severity of infection. Generally, ciprofloxacin should be continued for at least 2 days after the signs and symptoms of infection have disappeared. The usual duration is 7 to 14 days. Bone and joint infections may require treatment for 4 to 6 weeks or longer.

Ciprofloxacin hydrochloride tablets (Cipro®) for oral administration are available. Parenteral therapy may be changed to oral Cipro® tablets when the condition warrants, at the discretion of the physician. For complete dosage and administration information, see Cipro® tablet package insert.

Impaired Renal Function: The following table provides dosage guidelines for use in patients with renal impairment; however, monitoring of serum drug levels provides the most reliable basis for dosage adjustment.

RECOMMENDED STARTING AND MAINTENANCE DOSES FOR PATIENTS WITH IMPAIRED RENAL FUNCTION

Creatinine Clearance (mL/min)	Dosage
≥ 30	See usual dosage
5 – 29	200 – 400 mg q 18 – 24 hr

When only the serum creatinine concentration is known, the following formula may be used to estimate creatinine clearance.

$$\text{Men: Creatinine clearance (mL/min)} = \frac{\text{Weight (kg)} \times (140 - \text{age})}{72 \times \text{serum creatinine (mg/dL)}}$$

Women: $0.85 \times$ the value calculated for men.

The serum creatinine should represent a steady state of renal function.

For patients with changing renal function or for patients with renal impairment and hepatic insufficiency, measurement of serum concentrations of ciprofloxacin will provide additional guidance for adjusting dosage.

INTRAVENOUS ADMINISTRATION

Cipro® I.V. should be administered by intravenous infusion over a period of 60 minutes. Slow infusion of a dilute solution into a large vein will minimize patient discomfort and reduce the risk of venous irritation.

Vials (Injection Concentrate): THIS PREPARATION MUST BE DILUTED BEFORE USE. The intravenous dose should be prepared by aseptically withdrawing the appropriate volume of concentrate from the vials of Cipro® I.V. This should be diluted with a suitable intravenous solution to a final concentration of 1–2 mg/mL. (See COMPATIBILITY AND STABILITY.) The resulting solution should be infused over a period of 60 minutes by direct infusion or through a Y-type intravenous infusion set which may already be in place.

If this method or the "piggyback" method of administration is used, it is advisable to discontinue temporarily the administration of any other solutions during the infusion of Cipro® I.V.

Flexible Containers: Cipro® I.V. is also available as a 0.2% premixed solution in 5% dextrose in flexible containers of 100 mL or 200 mL. The solutions in flexible containers may be infused as described above.

COMPATIBILITY AND STABILITY

Ciprofloxacin injection 1% (10 mg/mL), when diluted with the following intravenous solutions to concentrations of 0.5 to 2.0 mg/mL, is stable for up to 14 days at refrigerated or room temperature storage.

0.9% Sodium Chloride Injection, USP
5% Dextrose Injection, USP

If Cipro® I.V. is to be given concomitantly with another drug, each drug should be given separately in accordance with the recommended dosage and route of administration for each drug.

HOW SUPPLIED

Cipro® I.V. (ciprofloxacin) is available as a clear, colorless to slightly yellowish solution. Cipro® I.V. is available in 200 mg and 400 mg strengths. The concentrate is supplied in vials while the premixed solution is supplied in flexible containers as follows:

CONTAINER	SIZE	STRENGTH	NDC NUMBER
Vial:	20mL	200 mg, 1%	0026-8562-20
	40mL	400 mg, 1%	0026-8564-64
Flexible Container:	100mL 5% dextrose	200 mg, 0.2%	0026-8552-36
	200mL 5% dextrose	400 mg, 0.2%	0026-8554-63

STORAGE

Vials:	Store between 41 – 77°F (5 – 25°C).
Flexible Container:	Store between 41 – 77°F (5 – 25°C).

Protect from light, avoid excessive heat, protect from freezing.

Ciprofloxacin is also available as Cipro® (ciprofloxacin HCl) Tablets 250, 500 and 750 mg.

ANIMAL PHARMACOLOGY

Ciprofloxacin and other quinolones have been shown to cause arthropathy in immature animals of most species tested. (See WARNINGS.) Damage of weight-bearing joints was observed in juvenile dogs and rats. In young beagles, 100 mg/kg ciprofloxacin given daily for 4 weeks caused degenerative articular changes of the knee joint. At 30 mg/kg, the effect on the joint was minimal. In a subsequent study in beagles, removal of weight-bearing from the joint reduced the lesions but did not totally prevent them.

Crystalluria, sometimes associated with secondary nephropathy, occurs in laboratory animals dosed with ciprofloxacin. This is primarily related to the reduced solubility of ciprofloxacin under alkaline conditions, which predominate in the urine of test animals; in man, crystalluria is rare since human urine is typically acidic. In rhesus monkeys, crystalluria without nephropathy has been noted after intravenous doses as low as 5 mg/kg. After 6 months of intravenous dosing at 10 mg/kg/day, no nephropathological changes were noted; however, nephropathy was observed after dosing at 20 mg/kg/day for the same duration.

In dogs, ciprofloxacin administered at 3 and 10 mg/kg by rapid intravenous injection (15 sec.) produces pronounced hypotensive effects. These effects are considered to be related to histamine release because they are partially antagonized by pyrilamine, an antihistamine. In rhesus monkeys, rapid intravenous injection also produces hypotension, but the effect in this species is inconsistent and less pronounced.

In mice, concomitant administration of nonsteroidal anti-inflammatory drugs, such as fenbufen, phenylbutazone and indomethacin, with quinolones has been reported to enhance the CNS stimulatory effect of quinolones.

Ocular toxicity, seen with some related drugs, has not been observed in ciprofloxacin-treated animals.

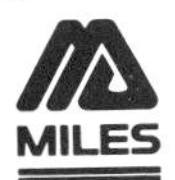

Miles Inc.
Pharmaceutical Division
400 Morgan Lane
West Haven, CT 06516 USA

Caution: Federal (USA) Law prohibits dispensing without a prescription.

PZ100736 9/91 BAY q 3939 5202-4-A-U.S.-1 1628
06-4745 Printed In U.S.A.

References: **1.** Phillips I, King A. Comparative activity of the 4-quinolones. *Rev Infect Dis.* 1988;10(suppl 1):S70-S76. **2.** Auckenthaler R, Michéa-Hamzehpour M, Pechère JC. *In-vitro* activity of newer quinolones against aerobic bacteria. *J Antimicrob Chemother.* 1986;17(suppl B):29-39. **3.** Pernet A. Temafloxacin overview. In: *Temafloxacin: A New Standard in Quinolones.* New York, NY: AVMD Group; 1990:1-13.

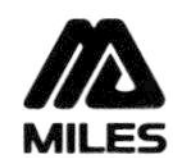

CIPRO®
(ciprofloxacin hydrochloride)
TABLETS

PZ100747

DESCRIPTION

Cipro® (ciprofloxacin hydrochloride) is a synthetic broad spectrum antibacterial agent for oral administration. Ciprofloxacin, a fluoroquinolone, is available as the monohydrochloride monohydrate salt of 1-cyclopropyl-6-fluoro-1, 4-dihydro-4-oxo-7-(1-piperazinyl)-3-quinolinecarboxylic acid. It is a faintly yellowish to light yellow crystalline substance with a molecular weight of 385.8. Its empirical formula is $C_{17}H_{18}FN_3O_3 \cdot HCl \cdot H_2O$ and its chemical structure is as follows:

Cipro® is available in 250 mg, 500 mg and 750 mg (ciprofloxacin equivalent) film-coated tablets. The inactive ingredients are starch, microcrystalline cellulose, silicon dioxide, crospovidone, magnesium stearate, hydroxypropyl methylcellulose, titanium dioxide, polyethylene glycol and water. Ciprofloxacin differs from other quinolones in that it has a fluorine atom at the 6-position, a piperazine moiety at the 7-position, and a cyclopropyl ring at the 1-position.

CLINICAL PHARMACOLOGY

Cipro® tablets are rapidly and well absorbed from the gastrointestinal tract after oral administration. The absolute bioavailability is approximately 70% with no substantial loss by first pass metabolism. Serum concentrations increase proportionally with the dose as shown:

Dose (mg)	Maximum Serum Concentration (µg/mL)	Area Under Curve (AUC) (µg • hr/mL)
250	1.2	4.8
500	2.4	11.6
750	4.3	20.2
1000	5.4	30.8

Maximum serum concentrations are attained 1 to 2 hours after oral dosing. Mean concentrations 12 hours after dosing with 250, 500, or 750 mg are 0.1, 0.2, and 0.4 µg/mL, respectively. The serum elimination half-life in subjects with normal renal function is approximately 4 hours.

Approximately 40 to 50% of an orally administered dose is excreted in the urine as unchanged drug. After a 250 mg oral dose, urine concentrations of ciprofloxacin usually exceed 200 µg/mL during the first two hours and are approximately 30 µg/mL at 8 to 12 hours after dosing. The urinary excretion of ciprofloxacin is virtually complete within 24 hours after dosing. The renal clearance of ciprofloxacin, which is approximately 300 mL/minute, exceeds the normal glomerular filtration rate of 120 mL/minute. Thus, active tubular secretion would seem to play a significant role in its elimination. Co-administration of probenecid with ciprofloxacin results in about a 50% reduction in the ciprofloxacin renal clearance and a 50% increase in its concentration in the systemic circulation. Although bile concentrations of ciprofloxacin are several fold higher than serum concentrations after oral dosing, only a small amount of the dose administered is recovered from the bile as unchanged drug. An additional 1-2% of the dose is recovered from the bile in the form of metabolites. Approximately 20 to 35% of an oral dose is recovered from the feces within 5 days after dosing. This may arise from either biliary clearance or transintestinal elimination. Four metabolites have been identified in human urine which together account for approximately 15% of an oral dose. The metabolites have antimicrobial activity, but are less active than unchanged ciprofloxacin.

When Cipro® is given concomitantly with food, there is a delay in the absorption of the drug, resulting in peak concentrations that are closer to 2 hours after dosing rather than 1 hour. The overall absorption, however, is not substantially affected. Concurrent administration of antacids containing magnesium hydroxide or aluminum hydroxide may reduce the bioavailability of ciprofloxacin by as much as 90%. (See PRECAUTIONS.)

Concomitant administration of ciprofloxacin with theophylline decreases the clearance of theophylline resulting in elevated serum theophylline levels, and increased risk of a patient developing CNS or other adverse reactions. Ciprofloxacin also decreases caffeine clearance and inhibits the formation of paraxanthine after caffeine administration. (See PRECAUTIONS.)

In patients with reduced renal function, the half-life of ciprofloxacin is slightly prolonged. Dosage adjustments may be required. (See DOSAGE AND ADMINISTRATION.)

In preliminary studies in patients with stable chronic liver cirrhosis, no significant changes in ciprofloxacin pharmacokinetics have been observed. The kinetics of ciprofloxacin in patients with acute hepatic insufficiency, however, have not been fully elucidated.

The binding of ciprofloxacin to serum proteins is 20 to 40% which is not likely to be high enough to cause significant protein binding interactions with other drugs.

After oral administration ciprofloxacin is widely distributed throughout the body. Tissue concentrations often exceed serum concentrations in both men and women, particularly in genital tissue including the prostate. Ciprofloxacin is present in active form in the saliva, nasal and bronchial secretions, sputum, skin blister fluid, lymph, peritoneal fluid, bile and prostatic secretions. Ciprofloxacin has also been detected in lung, skin, fat, muscle, cartilage, and bone. The drug diffuses into the cerebrospinal fluid (CSF); however, CSF concentrations are generally less than 10% of peak serum concentrations. Low levels of the drug have been detected in the aqueous and vitreous humors of the eye.

Microbiology: Ciprofloxacin has *in vitro* activity against a wide range of gram-negative and gram-positive organisms. The bactericidal action of ciprofloxacin results from interference with the enzyme DNA gyrase which is needed for the synthesis of bacterial DNA.

Ciprofloxacin has been shown to be active against most strains of the following organisms both *in vitro* and in clinical infections (See INDICATIONS AND USAGE section):

Gram-positive bacteria

Enterococcus faecalis (Many strains are only moderately susceptible)
Staphylococcus aureus
Staphylococcus epidermidis
Streptococcus pneumoniae
Streptococcus pyogenes

Gram-negative bacteria

Campylobacter jejuni
Citrobacter diversus
Citrobacter freundii
Enterobacter cloacae
Escherichia coli
Haemophilus influenzae
Haemophilus parainfluenzae
Klebsiella pneumoniae
Morganella morganii
Proteus mirabilis
Proteus vulgaris
Providencia rettgeri
Providencia stuartii
Pseudomonas aeruginosa
Serratia marcescens
Shigella flexneri
Shigella sonnei

Ciprofloxacin has been shown to be active *in vitro* against most strains of the following organisms; however, *the clinical significance of these data is unknown.*

Gram-positive bacteria

Staphylococcus haemolyticus
Staphylococcus hominis
Staphylococcus saprophyticus

Gram-negative bacteria

Acinetobacter calcoaceticus subs. *anitrastus*
Acinetobacter calcoaceticus subs. *lwoffi*
Aeromonas caviae
Aeromonas hydrophila
Brucella melitensis
Campylobacter coli
Edwardsiella tarda
Enterobacter aerogenes
Haemophilus ducreyi
Klebsiella oxytoca
Legionella pneumophila
Moraxella (Branhamella) catarrhalis
Neisseria gonorrhoeae
Neisseria meningitidis
Pasteurella multocida
Salmonella enteritidis
Salmonella typhi
Vibrio cholerae
Vibrio parahaemolyticus
Vibrio vulnificus
Yersinia enterocolitica

Other organisms

Chlamydia trachomatis (only moderately susceptible)
Mycobacterium tuberculosis (only moderately susceptible)

Most strains of *Pseudomonas cepacia* and some strains of *Xanthomonas (Pseudomonas) maltophilia* are resistant to ciprofloxacin as are most anaerobic bacteria, including *Bacteroides fragilis* and *Clostridium difficile.*

Ciprofloxacin is slightly less active when tested at acidic pH. The inoculum size has little effect when tested *in vitro*. The minimum bactericidal concentration (MBC) generally does not exceed the minimum inhibitory concentration (MIC) by more than a factor of 2. Resistance to ciprofloxacin *in vitro* develops slowly (multiple-step mutation).

Ciprofloxacin does not cross-react with other antimicrobial agents such as beta-lactams or aminoglycosides; therefore, organisms resistant to these drugs may be susceptible to ciprofloxacin.

In vitro studies have shown that additive activity often results when ciprofloxacin is combined with other antimicrobial agents such as beta-lactams, aminoglycosides, clindamycin, or metronidazole. Synergy has been reported particularly with the combination of ciprofloxacin and a beta-lactam; antagonism is observed only rarely.

Susceptibility Tests

Diffusion Techniques: Quantitative methods that require measurement of zone diameters give the most precise estimates of susceptibility of bacteria to antimicrobial agents. One such standardized procedure[1] which has been recommended for use with disks to test susceptibility of organisms to ciprofloxacin uses the 5-µg ciprofloxacin disk. Interpretation involves correlation of the diameters obtained in the disk test with the minimum inhibitory concentrations (MICs) for ciprofloxacin.

Reports from the laboratory giving results of the standard single-disk susceptibility test with a 5-µg ciprofloxacin disk should be interpreted according to the following criteria:

Zone Diameter (mm)	Interpretation
≥ 21	(S) Susceptible
16 – 20	(I) Intermediate (Moderately Susceptible)
≤ 15	(R) Resistant

A report of "Susceptible" indicates that the pathogen is likely to be inhibited by generally achievable blood levels. A report of "Intermediate (Moderately Susceptible)" suggests that the organism would be susceptible if high dosage is used or if the infection is confined to tissues and fluids in which high antimicrobial levels are attained. A report of "Resistant" indicates that achievable drug concentrations are unlikely to be inhibitory and other therapy should be selected.

Dilution Techniques: Use a standardized dilution method[2] (broth, agar, microdilution) or equivalent with ciprofloxacin powder. The MIC values obtained should be interpreted according to the following criteria:

MIC (µg/mL)	Interpretation
≤ 1	(S) Susceptible
2	(I) Intermediate (Moderately Susceptible)
≥ 4	(R) Resistant

Standardized procedures require the use of laboratory control organisms. This is true for both standardized diffusion techniques and standardized dilution techniques. The 5-µg ciprofloxacin disk should give the following zone diameters and the standard ciprofloxacin powder should provide the following MIC values:

QC Strains	Disk Zone Diameter (mm)	MIC (µg/mL)
S. aureus (ATCC 25923)	22 – 30	—
S. aureus (ATCC 29213)	—	0.12 – 0.5
E. coli (ATCC 25922)	30 – 40	0.004 – 0.015
P. aeruginosa (ATCC 27853)	25 – 33	0.25 – 1.0
E. faecalis (ATCC 29212)	—	0.25 – 2.0

For anaerobic bacteria the MIC of ciprofloxacin can be determined by agar or broth dilution (including microdilution) techniques[3].

INDICATIONS AND USAGE

Cipro® is indicated for the treatment of infections caused by susceptible strains of the designated microorganisms in the conditions listed below. Please see DOSAGE AND ADMINISTRATION for specific recommendations.

Lower Respiratory Infections caused by *Escherichia coli, Klebsiella pneumoniae, Enterobacter cloacae, Proteus mirabilis, Pseudomonas aeruginosa, Haemophilus influenzae, Haemophilus parainfluenzae*, or *Streptococcus pneumoniae*.

Skin and Skin Structure Infections caused by *Escherichia coli, Klebsiella pneumoniae, Enterobacter cloacae, Proteus mirabilis, Proteus vulgaris, Providencia stuartii, Morganella morganii, Citrobacter freundii, Pseudomonas aeruginosa, Staphylococcus aureus, Staphylococcus epidermidis*, or *Streptococcus pyogenes*.

Bone and Joint Infections caused by *Enterobacter cloacae, Serratia marcescens*, or *Pseudomonas aeruginosa*.

Urinary Tract Infections caused by *Escherichia coli, Klebsiella pneumoniae, Enterobacter cloacae, Serratia marcescens, Proteus mirabilis, Providencia rettgeri, Morganella morganii, Citrobacter diversus, Citrobacter freundii, Pseudomonas aeruginosa, Staphylococcus epidermidis*, or *Enterococcus faecalis*.

Infectious Diarrhea caused by *Escherichia coli* (enterotoxigenic strains), *Campylobacter jejuni, Shigella flexneri** or *Shigella sonnei** when antibacterial therapy is indicated.

*Although treatment of infections due to this organism in this organ system demonstrated a clinically significant outcome, efficacy was studied in fewer than 10 patients.

If anaerobic organisms are suspected of contributing to the infection, appropriate therapy should be administered.

Appropriate culture and susceptibility tests should be performed before treatment in order to isolate and identify organisms causing infection and to determine their susceptibility to ciprofloxacin. Therapy with Cipro® may be initiated before results of these tests are known; once results become available appropriate therapy should be continued. As with other drugs, some strains of *Pseudomonas aeruginosa* may develop resistance fairly rapidly during treatment with ciprofloxacin. Culture and susceptibility testing performed periodically during therapy will provide information not only on the therapeutic effect of the antimicrobial agent but also on the possible emergence of bacterial resistance.

CONTRAINDICATIONS

Cipro® (ciprofloxacin hydrochloride) is contraindicated in persons with a history of hypersensitivity to ciprofloxacin or any member of the quinolone class of antimicrobial agents.

WARNINGS

THE SAFETY AND EFFECTIVENESS OF CIPROFLOXACIN IN CHILDREN, ADOLESCENTS (LESS THAN 18 YEARS OF AGE), PREGNANT WOMEN, AND LACTATING WOMEN HAVE NOT BEEN ESTABLISHED. (SEE PRECAUTIONS-PEDIATRIC USE, PREGNANCY AND NURSING MOTHERS SUBSECTIONS.) The oral administration of ciprofloxacin caused lameness in immature dogs. Histopathological examination of the weight-bearing joints of these dogs revealed permanent lesions of the cartilage. Related quinolone-class drugs also produce erosions of cartilage of weight-bearing joints and other signs of arthropathy in immature animals of various species. (See ANIMAL PHARMACOLOGY.)

Convulsions have been reported in patients receiving ciprofloxacin. Convulsions, increased intracranial pressure, and toxic psychosis have been reported in patients receiving drugs in this class. Quinolones may also cause central nervous system (CNS) stimulation which may lead to tremors, restlessness, lightheadedness, confusion and hallucinations. If these reactions occur in patients receiving ciprofloxacin, the drug should be discontinued and appropriate measures instituted. As with all quinolones, ciprofloxacin should be used with caution in patients with known or suspected CNS disorders, such as severe cerebral arteriosclerosis, epilepsy, and other factors that predispose to seizures. (See ADVERSE REACTIONS.)

SERIOUS AND FATAL REACTIONS HAVE BEEN REPORTED IN PATIENTS RECEIVING CONCURRENT ADMINISTRATION OF CIPROFLOXACIN AND THEOPHYLLINE. These reactions have included cardiac arrest, seizure, status epilepticus and respiratory failure. Although similar serious adverse events have been reported in patients receiving theophylline alone, the possibility that these reactions may be potentiated by ciprofloxacin cannot be eliminated. If concomitant use cannot be avoided, serum levels of theophylline should be monitored and dosage adjustments made as appropriate.

Serious and occasionally fatal hypersensitivity (anaphylactic) reactions, some following the first dose, have been reported in patients receiving quinolone therapy. Some reactions were accompanied by cardiovascular collapse, loss of consciousness, tingling, pharyngeal or facial edema, dyspnea, urticaria, and itching. Only a few patients had a history of hypersensitivity reactions. Serious anaphylactic reactions require immediate emergency treatment with epinephrine. Oxygen, intravenous steroids, and airway management, including intubation, should be administered as indicated.

Severe hypersensitivity reactions characterized by rash, fever, eosinophilia, jaundice, and hepatic necrosis with fatal outcome have also been rarely reported in patients receiving ciprofloxacin along with other drugs. The possibility that these reactions were related to ciprofloxacin cannot be excluded. Ciprofloxacin should be discontinued at the first appearance of a skin rash or any other sign of hypersensitivity.

Pseudomembranous colitis has been reported with nearly all antibacterial agents, including ciprofloxacin, and may range in severity from mild to life-threatening. Therefore, it is important to consider this diagnosis in patients who present with diarrhea subsequent to the administration of antibacterial agents.

Treatment with antibacterial agents alters the normal flora of the colon and may permit overgrowth of clostridia. Studies indicate that a toxin produced by *Clostridium difficile* is one primary cause of "antibiotic-associated colitis".

After the diagnosis of pseudomembranous colitis has been established, therapeutic measures should be initiated. Mild cases of pseudomembranous colitis usually respond to drug discontinuation alone. In moderate to severe cases, consideration should be given to management with fluids and electrolytes, protein supplementation and treatment with an antibacterial drug clinically effective against *C. difficile* colitis.

PRECAUTIONS

General: Crystals of ciprofloxacin have been observed rarely in the urine of human subjects but more frequently in the urine of laboratory animals, which is usually alkaline. (See ANIMAL PHARMACOLOGY.) Crystalluria related to ciprofloxacin has been reported only rarely in humans because human urine is usually acidic. Alkalinity of the urine should be avoided in patients receiving ciprofloxacin. Patients should be well hydrated to prevent the formation of highly concentrated urine.

Alteration of the dosage regimen is necessary for patients with impairment of renal function. (See DOSAGE AND ADMINISTRATION.)

Moderate to severe phototoxicity manifested by an exaggerated sunburn reaction has been observed in patients who are exposed to direct sunlight while receiving some members of the quinolone class of drugs. Excessive sunlight should be avoided. Therapy should be discontinued if phototoxicity occurs.

As with any potent drug, periodic assessment of organ system functions, including renal, hepatic, and hematopoietic function, is advisable during prolonged therapy.

Information for Patients: Patients should be advised that ciprofloxacin may be taken with or without meals. The preferred time of dosing is two hours after a meal. Patients should also be advised to drink fluids liberally and not take antacids containing magnesium, aluminum, or calcium, products containing iron, or multivitamins containing zinc. However, usual dietary intake of calcium has not been shown to alter the absorption of ciprofloxacin.

Patients should be advised that ciprofloxacin may be associated with hypersensitivity reactions, even following a single dose, and to discontinue the drug at the first sign of a skin rash or other allergic reaction.

Patients should be advised to avoid excessive sunlight or artificial ultraviolet light while receiving ciprofloxacin and to discontinue therapy if phototoxicity occurs.

Ciprofloxacin may cause dizziness and lightheadedness; therefore patients should know how they react to this drug before they operate an automobile or machinery or engage in activities requiring mental alertness or coordination.

Patients should be advised that ciprofloxacin may increase the effects of theophylline and caffeine. There is a possibility of caffeine accumulation when products containing caffeine are consumed while taking quinolones.

Drug Interactions: As with some other quinolones, concurrent administration of ciprofloxacin with theophylline may lead to elevated serum concentrations of theophylline and prolongation of its elimination half-life. This may result in increased risk of theophylline-related adverse reactions. (See WARNINGS.) If concomitant use cannot be avoided, serum levels of theophylline should be monitored and dosage adjustments made as appropriate.

Some quinolones, including ciprofloxacin, have also been shown to interfere with the metabolism of caffeine. This may lead to reduced clearance of caffeine and a prolongation of its serum half-life.

Concurrent administration of ciprofloxacin with antacids containing magnesium, aluminum, or calcium; with sucralfate or divalent and trivalent cations such as iron may substantially interfere with the absorption of ciprofloxacin, resulting in serum and urine levels considerably lower than desired. To a lesser extent this effect is demonstrated with zinc-containing multivitamins. (See DOSAGE AND ADMINISTRATION for concurrent administration of these agents with ciprofloxacin.)

Some quinolones, including ciprofloxacin, have been associated with transient elevations in serum creatinine in patients receiving cyclosporine concomitantly.

Quinolones have been reported to enhance the effects of the oral anticoagulant warfarin or its derivatives. When these products are administered concomitantly, prothrombin time or other suitable coagulation tests should be closely monitored.

Probenecid interferes with renal tubular secretion of ciprofloxacin and produces an increase in the level of ciprofloxacin in the serum. This should be considered if patients are receiving both drugs concomitantly.

As with other broad spectrum antimicrobial agents, prolonged use of ciprofloxacin may result in overgrowth of nonsusceptible organisms. Repeated evaluation of the patient's condition and microbial susceptibility testing is essential. If superinfection occurs during therapy, appropriate measures should be taken.

Carcinogenesis, Mutagenesis, Impairment of Fertility: Eight *in vitro* mutagenicity tests have been conducted with ciprofloxacin and the test results are listed below:

Salmonella/Microsome Test (Negative)
E. coli DNA Repair Assay (Negative)
Mouse Lymphoma Cell Forward Mutation Assay (Positive)
Chinese Hamster V_{79} Cell HGPRT Test (Negative)
Syrian Hamster Embryo Cell Transformation Assay (Negative)
Saccharomyces cerevisiae Point Mutation Assay (Negative)
Saccharomyces cerevisiae Mitotic Crossover and Gene Conversion Assay (Negative)
Rat Hepatocyte DNA Repair Assay (Positive)

Thus 2 of the 8 tests were positive but results of the following 3 *in vivo* test systems gave negative results:

Rat Hepatocyte DNA Repair Assay
Micronucleus Test (Mice)
Dominant Lethal Test (Mice)

Long term carcinogenicity studies in mice and rats have been completed. After daily oral dosing for up to 2 years, there is no evidence that ciprofloxacin had any carcinogenic or tumorigenic effects in these species.

Pregnancy: Teratogenic Effects. Pregnancy Category C: Reproduction studies have been performed in rats and mice at doses up to 6 times the usual daily human dose and have revealed no evidence of impaired fertility or harm to the fetus due to ciprofloxacin. In rabbits, as with most antimicrobial agents, ciprofloxacin (30 and 100 mg/kg orally) produced gastrointestinal disturbances resulting in maternal weight loss and an increased incidence of abortion. No teratogenicity was observed at either dose. After intravenous administration, at doses up to 20 mg/kg, no maternal toxicity was produced, and no embryotoxicity or teratogenicity was observed. There are, however, no adequate and well-controlled studies in pregnant women. Ciprofloxacin should be used during pregnancy only if the potential benefit justifies the potential risk to the fetus. (See WARNINGS.)

Nursing Mothers: Ciprofloxacin is excreted in human milk. Because of the potential for serious adverse reactions in infants nursing from mothers taking ciprofloxacin, a decision should be made either to discontinue nursing or to discontinue the drug, taking into account the importance of the drug to the mother.

Pediatric Use: Safety and effectiveness in children and adolescents less than 18 years of age have not been established. Ciprofloxacin causes arthropathy in juvenile animals. (See WARNINGS.)

ADVERSE REACTIONS

During clinical investigation, 2,799 patients received 2,868 courses of the drug. Adverse events that were considered likely to be drug related occurred in 7.3% of patients treated, possibly related in 9.2% (total of 16.5% thought to be possibly or probably related to drug therapy), and remotely related in 3.0%. Ciprofloxacin was discontinued because of an adverse event in 3.5% of patients treated, primarily involving the gastrointestinal system (1.5%), skin (0.6%), and central nervous system (0.4%).

The most frequently reported events, drug related or not, were nausea (5.2%), diarrhea (2.3%), vomiting (2.0%), abdominal pain/discomfort (1.7%), headache (1.2%), restlessness (1.1%), and rash (1.1%).

Additional events that occurred in less than 1% of ciprofloxacin treated patients are listed below.

CARDIOVASCULAR: palpitation, atrial flutter, ventricular ectopy, syncope, hypertension, angina pectoris, myocardial infarction, cardiopulmonary arrest, cerebral thrombosis

CENTRAL NERVOUS SYSTEM: dizziness, lightheadedness, insomnia, nightmares, hallucinations, manic reaction, irritability, tremor, ataxia, convulsive seizures, lethargy, drowsiness, weakness, malaise, anorexia, phobia, depersonalization, depression, paresthesia (See above.) (See PRECAUTIONS.)

GASTROINTESTINAL: painful oral mucosa, oral candidiasis, dysphagia, intestinal perforation, gastrointestinal bleeding (See above.) Cholestatic jaundice has been reported.

MUSCULOSKELETAL: joint or back pain, joint stiffness, achiness, neck or chest pain, flare up of gout

RENAL/UROGENITAL: interstitial nephritis, nephritis, renal failure, polyuria, urinary retention, urethral bleeding, vaginitis, acidosis

RESPIRATORY: dyspnea, epistaxis, laryngeal or pulmonary edema, hiccough, hemoptysis, bronchospasm, pulmonary embolism

SKIN/HYPERSENSITIVITY: pruritus, urticaria, photosensitivity, flushing, fever, chills, angioedema, edema of the face, neck, lips, conjunctivae or hands, cutaneous candidiasis, hyperpigmentation, erythema nodosum (See above.)

Allergic reactions ranging from urticaria to anaphylactic reactions have been reported. (See WARNINGS.)

SPECIAL SENSES: blurred vision, disturbed vision (change in color perception, overbrightness of lights), decreased visual acuity, diplopia, eye pain, tinnitus, hearing loss, bad taste

Most of the adverse events reported were described as only mild or moderate in severity, abated soon after the drug was discontinued, and required no treatment.

In several instances nausea, vomiting, tremor, irritability or palpitation were judged by investigators to be related to elevated serum levels of theophylline possibly as a result of drug interaction with ciprofloxacin.

Other adverse events reported in the postmarketing phase include anaphylactic reactions, erythema multiforme/Stevens-Johnson syndrome, exfoliative dermatitis, toxic epidermal necrolysis, vasculitis, jaundice, hepatic necrosis, toxic psychosis, postural hypotension, possible exacerbation of myasthenia gravis, anosmia, confusion, dysphasia, nystagmus, pseudomembranous colitis, pancreatitis, dyspepsia, flatulence, and constipation. Also reported were hemolytic anemia; agranulocytosis; elevation of serum triglycerides, serum cholesterol, blood glucose, serum potassium; prolongation of prothrombin time; albuminuria; candiduria, vaginal candidiasis; renal calculi; and change in serum phenytoin. (See PRECAUTIONS.)

Adverse Laboratory Changes: Changes in laboratory parameters listed as adverse events without regard to drug relationship:

Hepatic	— Elevations of: ALT (SGPT) (1.9%), AST (SGOT) (1.7%), alkaline phosphatase (0.8%), LDH (0.4%), serum bilirubin (0.3%).
Hematologic	— Eosinophilia (0.6%), leukopenia (0.4%), decreased blood platelets (0.1%), elevated blood platelets (0.1%), pancytopenia (0.1%).
Renal	— Elevations of: Serum creatinine (1.1%), BUN (0.9%). CRYSTALLURIA, CYLINDRURIA AND HEMATURIA HAVE BEEN REPORTED.

Other changes occurring in less than 0.1% of patients treated were: Elevation of serum gammaglutamyl transferase, elevation of serum amylase, reduction in blood glucose, elevated uric acid, decrease in hemoglobin, anemia, bleeding diathesis, increase in blood monocytes, leukocytosis.

OVERDOSAGE

In the event of acute overdosage, the stomach should be emptied by inducing vomiting or by gastric lavage. The patient should be carefully observed and given supportive treatment. Adequate hydration must be maintained. Only a small amount of ciprofloxacin (<10%) is removed from the body after hemodialysis or peritoneal dialysis.

DOSAGE AND ADMINISTRATION

The usual adult dosage for patients with urinary tract infections is 250 mg every 12 hours. For patients with complicated infections caused by organisms not highly susceptible, 500 mg may be administered every 12 hours.

Lower respiratory tract infections, skin and skin structure infections, and bone and joint infections may be treated with 500 mg every 12 hours. For more severe or complicated infections, a dosage of 750 mg may be given every 12 hours.

The recommended dosage for Infectious Diarrhea is 500 mg every 12 hours.

DOSAGE GUIDELINES

Location of Infection	Type or Severity	Unit Dose	Frequency	Daily Dose
Urinary tract	Mild/Moderate	250 mg	q 12 h	500 mg
	Severe/Complicated	500 mg	q 12 h	1000 mg
Lower respiratory tract;	Mild/Moderate	500 mg	q 12 h	1000 mg
Bone and Joint;	Severe/Complicated	750 mg	q 12 h	1500 mg
Skin or Skin Structure				
Infectious Diarrhea	Mild/Moderate/Severe	500 mg	q 12 h	1000 mg

The determination of dosage for any particular patient must take into consideration the severity and nature of the infection, the susceptibility of the causative organism, the integrity of the patient's host-defense mechanisms, and the status of renal function and hepatic function.

The duration of treatment depends upon the severity of infection. Generally ciprofloxacin should be continued for at least 2 days after the signs and symptoms of infection have disappeared. The usual duration is 7 to 14 days; however, for severe and complicated infections more prolonged therapy may be required. Bone and joint infections may require treatment for 4 to 6 weeks or longer. Infectious Diarrhea may be treated for 5-7 days.

Concurrent Use With Antacids or Multivalent Cations: Concurrent administration of ciprofloxacin with sucralfate or divalent and trivalent cations such as iron or antacids containing magnesium, aluminum, or calcium may substantially interfere with the absorption of ciprofloxacin, resulting in serum and urine levels considerably lower than desired. Therefore, concurrent administration of these agents with ciprofloxacin should be avoided. However, usual dietary intake of calcium has not been shown to alter the bioavailability of ciprofloxacin. Single dose bioavailability studies have shown that antacids may be administered either 2 hours after or 6 hours before ciprofloxacin dosing without a significant decrease in bioavailability. Histamine H_2-receptor antagonists appear to have no significant effect on the bioavailability of ciprofloxacin.

Impaired Renal Function: Ciprofloxacin is eliminated primarily by renal excretion; however, the drug is also metabolized and partially cleared through the biliary system of the liver and through the intestine. These alternate pathways of drug elimination appear to compensate for the reduced renal excretion in patients with renal impairment. Nonetheless, some modification of dosage is recommended, particularly for patients with severe renal dysfunction. The following table provides dosage guidelines for use in patients with renal impairment; however, monitoring of serum drug levels provides the most reliable basis for dosage adjustment:

RECOMMENDED STARTING AND MAINTENANCE DOSES FOR PATIENTS WITH IMPAIRED RENAL FUNCTION

Creatinine Clearance (mL/min)	Dose
> 50	See Usual Dosage
30 – 50	250 – 500 mg q 12 h
5 – 29	250 – 500 mg q 18 h
Patients on hemodialysis or Peritoneal dialysis	250 – 500 mg q 24 h (after dialysis)

When only the serum creatinine concentration is known, the following formula may be used to estimate creatinine clearance.

$$\text{Men: Creatinine clearance (mL/min)} = \frac{\text{Weight (kg)} \times (140 - \text{age})}{72 \times \text{serum creatinine (mg/dL)}}$$

Women: 0.85 × the value calculated for men.

The serum creatinine should represent a steady state of renal function.

In patients with severe infections and severe renal impairment, a unit dose of 750 mg may be administered at the intervals noted above; however, patients should be carefully monitored and the serum ciprofloxacin concentration should be measured periodically. Peak concentrations (1-2 hours after dosing) should generally range from 2 to 4 μg/mL.

For patients with changing renal function or for patients with renal impairment and hepatic insufficiency, measurement of serum concentrations of ciprofloxacin will provide additional guidance for adjusting dosage.

HOW SUPPLIED

Cipro® (ciprofloxacin hydrochloride) is available as round, slightly yellowish film-coated tablets containing 250 mg ciprofloxacin. The 250 mg tablet is coded with the word "Miles" on one side and "512" on the reverse side. Cipro® is also available as capsule shaped, slightly yellowish film-coated tablets containing 500 mg or 750 mg ciprofloxacin. The 500 mg tablet is coded with the word "Miles" on one side and "513" on the reverse side; the 750 mg tablet is coded with the word "Miles" on one side and "514" on the reverse side. Available in bottles of 50's, 100's and in Unit Dose packages of 100.

	Strength	NDC Code	Tablet Identification
Bottles of 50:	750 mg	NDC 0026-8514-50	Miles 514
Bottles of 100:	250 mg	NDC 0026-8512-51	Miles 512
	500 mg	NDC 0026-8513-51	Miles 513
Unit Dose Package of 100:	250 mg	NDC 0026-8512-48	Miles 512
	500 mg	NDC 0026-8513-48	Miles 513
	750 mg	NDC 0026-8514-48	Miles 514

Store below 86°F (30°C).

ANIMAL PHARMACOLOGY

Ciprofloxacin and other quinolones have been shown to cause arthropathy in immature animals of most species tested. (See WARNINGS.) Damage of weight bearing joints was observed in juvenile dogs and rats. In young beagles 100 mg/kg ciprofloxacin, given daily for 4 weeks, caused degenerative articular changes of the knee joint. At 30 mg/kg the effect on the joint was minimal. In a subsequent study in beagles removal of weight bearing from the joint reduced the lesions but did not totally prevent them.

Crystalluria, sometimes associated with secondary nephropathy, occurs in laboratory animals dosed with ciprofloxacin. This is primarily related to the reduced solubility of ciprofloxacin under alkaline conditions, which predominate in the urine of test animals; in man, crystalluria is rare since human urine is typically acidic. In rhesus monkeys, crystalluria without nephropathy has been noted after single oral doses as low as 5 mg/kg. After 6 months of intravenous dosing at 10 mg/kg/day, no nephropathological changes were noted; however, nephropathy was observed after dosing at 20 mg/kg/day for the same duration.

In dogs, ciprofloxacin at 3 and 10 mg/kg by rapid IV injection (15 sec.) produces pronounced hypotensive effects. These effects are considered to be related to histamine release since they are partially antagonized by pyrilamine, an antihistamine. In rhesus monkeys, rapid IV injection also produces hypotension but the effect in this species is inconsistent and less pronounced.

In mice, concomitant administration of nonsteroidal anti-inflammatory drugs such as fenbufen, phenylbutazone and indomethacin with quinolones has been reported to enhance the CNS stimulatory effect of quinolones.

Ocular toxicity seen with some related drugs has not been observed in ciprofloxacin-treated animals.

References: 1. National Committee for Clinical Laboratory Standards, Performance Standards for Antimicrobial Disk Susceptibility Tests-Fourth Edition. Approved Standard NCCLS Document M2-A4, Vol. 10, No. 7, NCCLS, Villanova, PA, April, 1990. **2.** National Committee for Clinical Laboratory Standards, Methods for Dilution Antimicrobial Susceptibility Tests for Bacteria that Grow Aerobically-Second Edition. Approved Standard NCCLS Document M7-A2, Vol. 10, No. 8, NCCLS, Villanova, PA, April, 1990. **3.** National Committee for Clinical Laboratory Standards, Methods for Antimicrobial Susceptiblity Testing of Anaerobic Bacteria-Second Edition. Approved Standard NCCLS Document M11-A2, Vol. 10, No. 15, NCCLS, Villanova, PA, December, 1990.

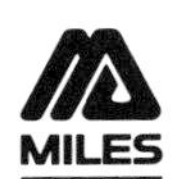

Miles Inc.
Pharmaceutical Division
400 Morgan Lane
West Haven, CT 06516 USA

Caution: Federal (USA) Law prohibits dispensing without a prescription.

PZ100747 1/93 Bay o 9867 2545 5202-2-A-U.S.-4 Printed in USA